Don't Kill the Birthday Girl

Don't Kill the Birthday Girl

TALES FROM AN ALLERGIC LIFE

· · · · · ·

SANDRA BEASLEY

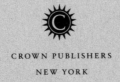

CROWN PUBLISHERS

NEW YORK

Library of Congress Cataloging-in-Publication Data
Beasley, Sandra.
Don't kill the birthday girl: tales from an allergic life/by Sandra Beasley.
p. cm.
1. Food allergy—United States—Case studies. 2. Beasley, Sandra—
Health. 3. Food allergy—Patients—United States—Biography. I. Title.
RC596.B425 2011
362.196′9750092—dc22
[B] 2010043724

ISBN 978-0-307-58811-1
eISBN 978-0-307-58813-5

PRINTED IN THE UNITED STATES OF AMERICA

Book design by Elizabeth Rendfleisch
Jacket design by Gabrielle Bordwin and Jean Traina
Jacket photography: Amana Productions Inc./Getty Images (cupcake);
Fuse/Getty Images (skull)

1 3 5 7 9 10 8 6 4 2

First Edition

For my mother,
who taught me the balancing act

$\cdot\cdot\cdot$ Contents $\cdot\cdot\cdot$

Don't Kill the Birthday Girl

There are only two birthdays that stand out in my memory as distinct, chronologically certain events. One: my sixteenth birthday, when we watched *Ferris Bueller's Day Off.* That was the year my friend Elizabeth, while using the swing anchored to the underside of our second-story deck, pushed off so hard that the whole shebang—girl, swing, unhooked chains—went sailing twenty feet out into the woods behind our house. Two: the year I got diagnosed with mononucleosis, too late to cancel an Italian-themed dinner party. So I stood in front of a stove for two hours—achy, glands swollen, stone-cold sober—cooking pasta for two dozen while my friends went through six bottles of wine. That was, undoubtedly, my twenty-first birthday.

Beyond that it blends into a murky ur-party. Which years did we go to Chuck E. Cheese's? When did I get my Rainbow Brite doll? Which years were my father home, and which years had the army sent him off to the War College, Saudi Arabia, Bosnia?

There is one constant in my birthday memories. When it came time for a cake, my mother would bring out whatever

Sandra-friendly sweet she'd designed. Some years it was sunflower-margarine Rice Krispies treats, and some years it was an applesauce-and-cinnamon-raisin bundt cake. I'd get my serving. Then we'd dish out the real dessert of cake or brownies or pie à la mode for everybody else. After singing, after blowing out candles, after presents had been opened, after everyone had eaten, someone would say it:

"Now, don't kill the birthday girl."

Which meant no kisses, no hugs, no touch of a hand or mouth. From that point onward, anyone who touched me ran the risk of giving me hives, or worse. Even today it's a phrase I repeat as part joke and part prayer.

Don't kill the birthday girl.

It's the same at every holiday. My uncle Jim is notorious for forgetting about my allergies, holding out a dish of ice cream and asking, "Want a bite?" He's the fun bachelor uncle, the one who rides a motorcycle and would give a little girl a windup sewer rat, complete with blinking red eyes, as a Christmas gift.

Once upon a time it would fall on my mother to protect me at the end of the night, when the aunts and uncles and cousins were making the rounds for good-byes. Now I step to the side on my own. Everyone understands why I avoid contact. Yet I can't help but wish it wasn't their last impression of me before the long drive home.

I am allergic to dairy (including goat's milk), egg, soy, beef, shrimp, pine nuts, cucumbers, cantaloupe, honeydew, mango, macadamias, pistachios, cashews, swordfish, and mustard. I'm also allergic to mold, dust, grass and tree pollen, cigarette smoke, dogs, rabbits, horses, and wool. But in particular, I am one of the more than 12 million Americans who has been di-agnosed with food allergies, a figure that includes almost 4 percent of all children. Even with so many of us in the conver-sation, there are huge disconnects in the dialogue. Parents who have never met a food they couldn't eat struggle to empathize with their child's allergies. Those crusading for community ac-commodation misguidedly conflate allergies with intolerance and confuse discomfort with anaphylaxis. Advocacy groups focus on youth allergies and largely ignore the complexities faced by those who grow into adulthood, travel, marry, and must figure out how to raise children of their own. There are multiple dimensions of data out there, but no one has set the gyroscope spinning.

Allergies are quirky beasts. Unlike many syndromes, they are primarily sorted according to their outside catalysts. (Have you ever heard someone claim to have type-peanut diabetes? Eggplant flu?) Allergies are widespread—and widely misdi-agnosed. There is a whole range of symptoms and degrees of sensitivity, and these symptoms can change for any given in-dividual at any time. For those with allergies like mine, each day requires vigilance in terms of what we do, the company we keep, and where we sit in relation to that bowl of mixed nuts. One person's comfort food is another person's enemy. One per-son's lifesaver is another's poison.

I thought my family's habit of calling the foods I can eat "Sandra-friendly" was unique, until I saw a book by Emily Hendrix called *Sophie-Safe Cooking: A Collection of Family Friendly Recipes That Are Free of Milk, Eggs, Wheat, Soy, Peanuts, Tree Nuts, Fish, and Shellfish*. The more I have read, the more I realize a whole culture of catchphrases has emerged in addition to the key medical terminology. "Safe," "friendly," "free": these words come up over and over again in literature about allergies.

Don't kill the birthday girl. Leftover omelet clings to the edge of a breakfast plate. Butter greases the stir-fry. Walnuts go commando in an otherwise tame brownie. There's a reason they're called allergy "attacks"; you never know where a food can be lurking.

But those with food allergies aren't victims. We're people who—for better or for worse—experience the world in a slightly different way. This is not a story of how we die. These are the stories of how we live.

CHAPTER ONE

I Am Jane's Anaphylactic Shock

In the early 1990s, many Americans were swept up by an interest in healthy eating. The U.S. Department of Agriculture began working on its Food Guide Pyramid, which would be released in 1992. When I first heard about this "pyramid" in fourth grade, I assumed it was based on the cuisine of Egyptians (blame the world history unit we had finished only a few days earlier). I imagined the pantries of ancient Cairo: fish, cakes of grain, honey, tiger nuts, and the occasional wayward canopic jar of kidneys.

My fourth-grade teacher invited a professional nutritionist, the mother of one of the other students, to come in for a lesson on maintaining a proper diet. She was a short, trim, olive-skinned woman with a clipped voice. She moved her pointer with enthusiastic precision over each part of her diagram, which presaged the portions that would be recommended by the USDA. She began by suggesting a soft, cushiony foundation of six to eleven servings of grains per day. This was in an era when Wonder bread and brown rice stood side by side as equals in the ranks of starch. Beans and beef, eggs and nuts—all were packed neatly into the same block of two to three servings of protein.

Three glasses of whole milk? Yep, according to her diagram, that was the way to go. She tapped her pointer against the pyramid's penultimate tier.

"Milk prevents osteoporosis," she intoned.

No one asked the obvious: What was osteoporosis? Instead, one of my classmates raised her hand. "What if you don't drink milk?" she asked.

"There's cheese, if you don't like the taste of milk," the nutritionist replied. "The important thing is your daily calcium intake."

"What if you can't eat cheese?"

The nutritionist paused. "You should eat eggs," she said.

"What if you can't eat eggs?" another kid asked.

I knew what they were getting at. Three days earlier had been a much-anticipated pizza party. I'd gone to the library instead, to avoid exposure, which had prompted an explanation of my long list of food allergies.

My classmate raised his hand. "What if you can't have beef? Or ice cream? Or pizza, not even if you pick the cheese off?"

"Well," the nutritionist said brightly. "That's not somebody designed to survive, now, is it?"

She continued on to "Fats, Oils & Sweets," as I slumped down in my chair.

That was then. Today, vegan parents are raising vegan kids in vegan households, proving that not only can you survive without dairy but you can also procreate and thrive. Dietary restrictions and allergies have gone mainstream. When I hear that at Disney World, children with gluten allergies can order the Mickey Mouse pancakes and know that there is a gluten-free mix available, I think, *Things are different now.*

Then again, when on a weekend road trip I stop in at a rural Friendly's and ask for something, anything, guaranteed free of milk, eggs, or lard—only to watch the waitress shrug helplessly—I'm not so sure.

"Cereal?" I ask.

"Cereal? We don't have that," she says. "Where did you find that on the menu? Oh, there. I see it. Huh. No. What about the hash browns?"

"Are they cooked on the same griddle as stuff that's buttered?"

"Well, it's one big flattop back there." She waits pointedly as I weigh the odds. "How 'bout some coffee?"

"Sure," I say. She brings it with a side of cream.

When I was born in 1980, the world was a small-town waitress: it didn't know what to do with me. Fussing and crying, I would not breast-feed. When my parents tried to give me formula instead, it ran right through me. My stools turned black from internal bleeding. Within my first month I was back at the doctor's office, underweight and jaundiced. That's when the testing began. Goat's milk? Just as bad. Soy milk? Couldn't keep it down.

The doctors sent me home with a diagnosis of a broad

spectrum of allergies, which wouldn't be further determined until I was a little older. As an infant, my immune system was too underdeveloped to exhibit a traditional, identifiable reaction.

"So we raised you on juice and water," my mother told me. "Apple juice, then pineapple juice with Neo-Calglucon added for calcium. Rice. Creamed chicken. And on your first birthday, you had your first appointment with Dr. Latkin. You wore a white dress with pink polka dots."

My parents lived in a little brick house on 10th Road in Arlington, Virginia. My father, Mike, worked at a law firm downtown. In the years since his tour in Vietnam, he'd taken to growing his sandy-blond hair defiantly long, cutting it only for periodic reserves-duty weekends at Fort Meade. My mother, Bobbie, was a brunette beauty, a painter and printmaker who rented studio space at the Arlington Arts Center.

They had waited five years after marrying to have me. Like other first-time parents, they were terrified by the responsibility of keeping me safe from the Big, Bad World. Unlike other parents, they had to deal with the fact that the Big, Bad World was particularly out to get me. Take the Biscuit Incident: On a trip through Nashville, after hours of driving with a squalling, hungry three-year-old, they checked into Opryland and tried to figure out how to quell my growling stomach. My father's plate came with a plain-looking biscuit on the side.

"You barely had *a crumb*," my mom said, still defensive after all these years. "We didn't know it was *buttermilk*." I began wheezing and hiving, spluttering at the liquid Benadryl they tried to ease down my throat. They waited, watching closely, unsure what to do. After an hour, I calmed down—probably as much from exhaustion as recovery—and fell asleep.

The next day my father was tied up in a conference, and my mother would not drive in an unfamiliar city. "The worst part was going back to that same hotel restaurant the next morning," she admitted, "and having to try again. We didn't know where else to take you."

By the time I was five, they recognized they had to instill absolute protective instincts. The traditional admonition of "Don't accept candy from strangers" became "Don't accept food—period." I tried to obey (and if I didn't, as my mother always points out, my body played tattletale). But sharing snacks is one of those critical gestures of friendship for the under-ten set, up there with trading bracelets or calling out someone's name during a game of Red Rover, Red Rover. It didn't take long before I phoned home from the nurse's office, dosed with Benadryl and snuffling through tears.

"It was just a potato chip," I said, mystified. "One potato chip!"

A sour-cream-flavored potato chip looked the same as the plain kind I ate all the time. How was it that I could react to something I couldn't even see? Working on a report for my third-grade class, I asked my allergist how the body recognized the invisible presence of milk.

"Imagine a workbench," Dr. Latkin said, "the kind with different-shaped holes for each block." I pictured my Fisher-Price toy at home, though that was baby stuff; I'd long since moved on to cultivating a collection of She-Ra action figures. The workbench, he explained, was like a kind of cell that could produce an allergic reaction.

"Now, you've got your blood," he said. "Little bits of food come floating down the bloodstream, like blocks." I nodded.

"If the shape of the block doesn't match the shape of the hole," he explained, "you won't have a reaction." But it didn't take much to change the shape of the block, he said. For example, cooked broccoli might have a different shape than raw broccoli. I visualized little crowns of broccoli bobbing along in my blood, a forest put out to sea.

"If the shape of the food matches the shape of the hole," he said, "your body tries to eliminate it." I remembered the red plastic hammer I had used to push each block through its hole. *Wham! Wham! Wham!*

"That's a reaction," he said.

I stared at him wide-eyed. No wonder I got all hivey. Somewhere inside me, I was being hit with a hammer.

It's not easy to explain allergies to a young child. My grasp of anatomy had a ways to go. This was also the age when I believed boogers were small, simple-minded animals that spent their lives roaming inside your nose, cleaning up whatever they found by eating it. To blow snot, I thought, with a twinge of guilt, was to kill one.

My classmates understood that my allergies made me different, though they weren't quite sure of the mechanics. They saw that I got out of sponge duty in the cafeteria (the slop water they used to wash down the tables was perpetually contaminated with milk). On the rare days I could buy Tater Tots, I was allowed to cut in the hot line rather than parade past all the stations I couldn't touch. Knowing I couldn't buy candy out of the on-site vending machines, my mother every day packed four or five strawberry candies—hard lozenges filled with jam—in my lunch bag, sugar capital that made me the kingpin of

Lunch Group B. In some ways, it seemed like "allergy girl" had a pretty sweet deal.

Thanks to my asthma, a frequent companion disease for allergies, when the other kids had to run the mile, I got to work the stopwatch and record times instead. One day my friend Karen crossed the finish line and let her forward momentum carry her into me, knocking us both down. The stopwatch and clipboard went flying. As we lay in a sprawled heap, she proceeded to rub her cheek against my forearms, over and over.

"What are you doing?" I asked, panting for breath.

"Whatever you are," she said, "I hope you're catching."

I had to have medications within quick reach. Since we were instructed to leave backpacks behind when traveling around school, I became the only kid at Haycock Elementary to carry a purse, the first of many hauled around over the years. There was the pink one with blue trim, an all-time favorite, ruined on a hot day at the funfair by a melted Jolly Rancher. There was LeSportsac, which I smugly informed my friends was "a French label." There was the black leather hand-me-down from my mother, still packed with musty, folded squares of Kleenex that bore lipstick blots.

Later in life, I would look on in awe at my friends' clutches and baguettes. I have never had a purse that wasn't wide enough for an EpiPen, deep enough for an inhaler, and complete with a zippered pocket for Benadryl. The plastic orange chairs used in our classrooms were not designed for purses. Their backrests had rounded-down corners that offered no resistance to gravity. So whenever I twitched or stretched in my seat, the purse would fall to the linoleum, necessitating a backward reach that made it look like I was trying to pass a note. Grab; hang; thunk. Grab; hang; thunk.

Picture a kid in thick-lensed glasses, indigo-dark jeans (my mother refused to buy "that worn-out stonewashed look"), a beglittered T-shirt threaded through a plastic buckle-loop that gave it an asymmetrical hem, and a slap bracelet. Now add the purse of a thirty-two-year-old mother, complete with pills, tissues, safety pins, and too many pennies. That is the hybrid reality of a child with food allergies.

I took refuge in books. My grandfather, a doctor, noticed my love of reading and began passing along his monthly *Reader's Digest* whenever I went to visit. I was fascinated by all the features ("Drama in Real Life," "Laughter, the Best Medicine," even that diabolical Word Power quiz), but my runaway favorite was "I am Joe's . . ."/"I am Jane's . . . ," a series written from the point of view of various body parts as they experienced critical injury or illness. The author, J. D. Ratcliff, assuming the voice of "Joe's back," had my full attention as he explained what it felt like to herniate, undergo a CT scan, and slip those little disks back into their proper lumbar positions.

I adored these columns partially because they satisfied my flair for the dramatic. Who *didn't* want Jane's thyroid, or Joe's lungs? Their viscera were so much more interesting than mine. Between the ages of eight and twelve, I was sure I had experienced bouts with kidney stones, obsessive-compulsive disorder, mammary cysts (which turned out to be . . . breasts), an arrhythmia, lockjaw, retinitis pigmentosa, and (though I was fuzzy on the details) prostate cancer.

There must have been days when my family regretted ever

introducing me to Joe and Jane. Perhaps they realized that in the long run, after my initial hypochondria passed, these articles would teach me the elements of diagnosis: developing internal measures of what was "normal" and what was aberrant, understanding how individual symptoms related to a whole, and knowing when to ask for help. In other words, these articles taught me how to manage allergic reactions. Preteens aren't known for their self-awareness, but I had no choice. No adult could do the job for me. Reactions that started out indiscernible to the outside world could turn quite serious. "I am Jane's funny-feeling throat" could transform, in a matter of minutes, to "I am Jane's anaphylactic shock."

. . .

A food becomes an allergen when the body decides to treat it as an enemy. The immune system creates a specific antibody designed to recognize each allergen. It's rare for someone to have an allergy attack the first time he or she tries a food. This can lead to a false sense of security among parents as they introduce new foods into their baby's diet. But it's the second time that's the charm—or in this case, the curse.

The newly minted antibody (usually the protein type immunoglobulin E, also called IgE), circulates through the bloodstream and attaches to the surface of mast cells. Mast cells can be found in virtually all body tissue but are particularly populous in the skin, nose, throat, lungs, and gastrointestinal tract—the places someone typically might feel an allergy attack. When a reaction occurs, IgE causes the mast cells to release a massive dose of chemicals (including histamine) called "mediators." That is a misleadingly innocuous term. They should be called "hit men."

If the affected mast cells are in the skin, lips, and eyelids, you get hives. If they are in the throat, you choke up and vomit. If they are in the lungs, you wheeze. You can imagine what havoc ensues in the GI tract. One measure of the severity of an allergy is a scale of 1 to 5; "level 5" indicates an extremely high antibody population in the bloodstream. The more IgE poised to respond, the more sensitive the patient is to even the smallest presence of the allergen and, in most cases, the more severe the reaction.

A level 5 allergy may trigger an anaphylactic reaction in which so many different vital functions shut down so fast that the body goes into shock. Blood pressure plummets and the patient loses consciousness. Anaphylaxis first grabbed pop culture's attention in the context of bee stings. (See exhibit A: Thomas J. in the 1991 movie *My Girl*. If your character is a quirky outsider with severe allergies, your days are numbered.)

I wish I could say that if five minutes have passed after exposure to an allergen and you are still upright, then you have dodged the bullet of anaphylaxis. But that's not the case. A reaction can start within seconds, or accumulate over a period of several hours. Some scientists believe delayed reactions result from a different antibody response—immunoglobulin G, or IgG—particularly primed to respond to such allergens as milk, wheat, and corn. After one ill-fated dinner party, I was awakened in the middle of the night by an attack I thought I'd tamed before going to bed, with a reaction much worse than the one

I'd had earlier. That's considered a biphasic reaction. In rare cases, anaphylaxis is triggered only if the allergen is combined with exercise in the three to four hours following exposure.

Anaphylactic reactions are sneaky bastards. On average they kill 150 people in America each year.

The eight most common food allergens in the United States are legally classified as milk, egg, peanuts, tree nuts, fish, shellfish, soy, and wheat. These foods account for more than 90 percent of allergies in the United States; there are about 160 known allergens, total. Corn and sesame are two other allergies with growing prevalence. Some of the least common food allergens are bananas, zucchini, potatoes, peas, turkey, and—though it seems exotic compared to the rest—avocado. All but avocado are popular in baby food form, and Gerber should probably get to work on a guacamole recipe.

The predisposition to develop allergies may be an inherited trait, but specific allergies are not. My father had allergies but outgrew almost all of them, which isn't happening in my case. He says that eating eggplant triggers an itchy throat, but we suspect this might be related to the fact that he detests eggplant. My mother experienced hives as a child, but she was never diagnosed with any specific food allergies. My younger sister doesn't have any food allergies except taro. Since her exposure took the form of tasting poi in Hawaii, she's not mourning the loss of taro from her diet.

There are a lot of gray areas in the realm of allergy. Celiac disease, often conflated with wheat allergy, is actually an autoimmune disorder of the small intestine that necessitates a gluten-free diet. But in acute cases, the severity of reaction demands zero tolerance for exposure—meaning those with celiac face the same attending social complications as those with deadly food allergies.

Then there are the widespread intolerances to food, most notably lactose. Too many times someone describes this as a "food allergy" when speaking with a waiter or host. It's not an allergy; it's a condition of missing enzymes, translating into an inability to digest milk sugar, which causes abdominal pain.

I confess that when someone claims to have a dairy allergy, then indulges in a chocolate-chip cookie because he or she is willing to tolerate bloating and stomachaches later in the day, I get annoyed. That kind of behavior makes us all less credible. There's a reason the food allergic have taken to using the phrase "true allergy." Millions of people have been diagnosed with food allergies. Yet the medical understanding of what causes them, and how to control or cure them, is maddeningly incomplete.

· · ·

The mystery of allergies has been around since antiquity. Between the sixth and fourth centuries BCE, a collective of physicians that included Hippocrates of Kos composed the sixty or so treatises known as the Hippocratic Corpus, rejecting superstition to treat medicine as a science. The Corpus is known for giving us the phrase "First do no harm," which is often conflated with the Hippocratic oath (though that exact phrase in translation is actually found in a different work of the Corpus, *Epidemics*).

Buried in this compendium of textbooks, lectures, and notes on philosophy is the observation that some patients can eat cheese "without the slightest hurt . . . [while] others come off badly." Many historians of science believe this to be the first recorded recognition of allergies. The larger passage makes clear that the cheese does not cause the suffering directly; the cheese is not spoiled or poisoned. Rather, that particular body exhibits a hardwired and self-destructive response, a "hostile humor" to cheese.

Subsequent generations of physicians were fascinated by this observation, but little research focused on the physiological roots of the phenomenon. Sir John Floyer, an English physician born in 1649, was one exception. He carefully listed the food, powders, and vapors that precipitated his asthmatic patients' difficulty in breathing.

That's not Floyer's claim to fame. He is remembered because he was the one who recommended to Sarah Ford—also known as Mrs. Michael Johnson—that she take her young son to the court of Queen Anne, where he would be touched and cured of the "King's Evil." This proved to be a seminal event in the life of a certain Samuel Johnson. In addition to shaping the life of that literary critic, Floyer invented a watch for the purpose of measuring pulse, which he believed was a key indicator of health. But as far as allergies went, well, there wasn't even a name for the phenomenon yet.

It wasn't until 1906 that Clemens von Pirquet, an Austrian doctor engaged in research on smallpox and tuberculosis, coined the term *allergie* or *allergy.* His conflation of Greek words for *other* and *energy* evoked his theory that the disparate arrays of symptoms—i.e., edema, hives, vomiting—that he had observed in experiments were, in fact, a coherent biological reaction coordinated through the immune system: a hypersensitivity to ingested foreign materials that increased with subsequent trials. Not all of his fellow scientists welcomed von Pirquet's insight. Quite the opposite. He started what would now be called a battle for brand recognition.

Prominent French physiologist Charles Richet publicly dismissed the word *allergy* on the grounds that the term he had created in 1902, *anaphylaxis* (rough translation: "absence of guard"), did a perfectly good job describing the issue. Richet would go on to win the 1913 Nobel Prize in Physiology or Medicine for his work with anaphylaxis, which he defined as any sensitivity developed in an organism after receiving an injection of a protein, colloid, or toxin. An expert on extrasensory perception and the occult, Richet's other coinages included *ectoplasm* and *metapsychics*. We can also thank him for figuring out that animals shiver in order to regulate body temperature.

For von Pirquet, this professional turf war was endemic of a career that always fell one step short of fame. Another French scientist, Charles Mantoux, used von Pirquet's research to develop an effective way of screening for tuberculosis infection. This procedure promptly became known as the Mantoux test. Five times von Pirquet would be nominated for the Nobel Prize, and five times he would not win.

Anaphylaxis captured the big picture of a body's shutdown response, and the word is still used today. But von Pirquet's work in the clinics of Austria—augmented by time spent in Paris and Baltimore, Maryland, where he was offered a professorship at Johns Hopkins—rightly focused not on the antigens of invading matter but on the antibodies of the host. His point that the greatest damage was host inflicted placed him in step with an important generation of physicians including Ludwik

Fleck and Carl Weigert (who called it the "Siva effect," invoking the self-sacrificing Hindu god). Many of our critical understandings of how allergic reactions form—only after the initial exposure, using an incubation period that shortens after subsequent exposures, and manifesting in a variety of symptoms for a variety of allergens—come from von Pirquet's findings.

By the 1920s, both the terms *allergy* and *anaphylaxis* were used in scholarly texts, and the former would eventually overtake the latter in public parlance. But professional success can't cure personal despair. In 1929, Clemens von Pirquet and his wife, Maria, committed suicide using cyanide. In his final years, the doctor had used sophisticated statistical analysis to identify correlations between volume of deaths and calendar date, laying the groundwork for what we can now identify as "seasonal" illnesses, such as hay fever. And depression.

Baron von Pirquet poisoned himself in February. Just nine months later, in November 1929, a new magazine debuted in America: *Journal of Allergy.*

Scientific interest in the allergy phenomenon had solidified under a common name, yet this did not translate to immediate medical comprehension. In the 1940s and early 1950s, physicians attributed illnesses as diverse as migraines, colitis, and multiple sclerosis to the villain of allergies. Allergies, together with hay fever and asthma, were the evil henchmen of increasing urbanization. Doctors prescribed "fresh air"; allergy sufferers were sent off to frolic in fields of ragweed. Magazine ads encouraged patients to light up a stramonium cigarette filled with jimsonweed, the dried hallucinogen also known as the devil's trumpet.

There were a few important technical and theoretical

advances during this time. Diphenhydramine, one of the first antihistamines, was invented by Cincinnati chemical engineer Dr. George Rieveschl in 1943 and approved by the Food and Drug Administration for prescription usage in 1946. Pfizer would later trademark the drug under the name Benadryl, and today it is available in a number of generic formats. Like-minded research in Europe led pharmaceutical companies to flood the market with antihistamines, which address allergic reactions directly by blocking histamine receptor sites. These are often paired with decongestant tablets that help manage attack symptoms.

Today, other available oral treatments include montelukast sodium, a leukotriene antagonist (meaning that it attacks other mediators of inflammation besides histamines) that is marketed under the name Singulair and is primarily used to treat chronic asthma. And in cases where a progressing attack interferes with the ability to swallow, a patient can use a nebulizer that converts a liquid medicine to an inhalable aerosol.

For the most acute attacks, a patient can self-administer a shot of epinephrine using an EpiPen or Twinject injector, to be followed by immediate medical care. Anyone who has been diagnosed with the potential for anaphylaxis is advised to carry an injector at all times. There's brisk business in carriers designed for the fashion savvy or, in the case of mothers buying for allergic sons, anything that doesn't resemble a tampon holder.

The 1940s also welcomed the first official "allergy clinic," established in London at St. Mary's Hospital and headed by John Freeman, who was a pioneer in the field of immunotherapy injections. Using pollen allergies as their model, Freeman and his colleague Leonard Noon theorized that regular subcutaneous doses of a known allergen administered in "Noon units," extracts measured in weight per milliliter, could desensitize the patient. Today, shots are an FDA-approved therapy for allergies to pollen, pet dander, and insect stings. I collected approximately 782 I GOT MY SHOT TODAY stickers over time, including a complete series featuring the members of New Kids on the Block. Though they have never proven particularly successful at reducing food sensitivity, and some experts doubt their overall effectiveness, they remain one of the most popular forms of treatment for children with allergies.

Much has changed in sixty years; much remains the same. A patient walking into St. Mary's in 1946 might have received, essentially, the same prick test I would have received in 1986. The prick test is as elegant a diagnostic tool as one would suspect given its name. A technician uses a lancet to create a grid of tiny subcutaneous breaks in the skin of the subject's back or forearm. Each prick point is then swabbed with the essence of one of the allergens being tested. After an appropriate waiting period, the skin is inspected for skin rash, hives, or other reaction. The bigger the wheal, the worse the allergy, but the nature of delivery ensures a reaction usually no more serious than a mosquito bite.

Like some of the simplest antihistamine compounds, this procedure endures in the modern day because it is easily available, is comparatively inexpensive, and provides fast results. But it's also traumatic. There's nothing worse than lying on your belly feeling a fiery swelling as it spreads across your back and being forbidden to scratch the itch, while a doctor says, "'My goodness, look at that. That there.'"

Giving patients the option of a less visceral diagnostic process, in 1974, a Swedish laboratory trademarked the RAST (radioallergosorbent test), which surveys a blood sample for the presence of specific immunoglobulin E antibodies. The yield of numeric data indicated not only the presence of allergies but also their severity, leading scientists to develop the rubric of level 1, level 2, and so on, assigned in correspondence to IgE frequency. Though RAST testing is expensive, it is now a standard diagnostic for those patients with a demonstrated capacity for anaphylactic reaction or with other factors that would complicate a skin test, such as eczema. The problem is that RAST testing, while useful, generates a lot of false positives. One of my rounds of RAST testing claimed I was allergic to both rice and pineapple—staple foods that have never caused a reaction when I've eaten them.

Ultimately, food allergies can be confirmed only with an oral food challenge. This is a fancy way of saying that you eat a teeny-tiny amount of the food, and you see what happens. There is a protocol for treating food challenges as a medical procedure: a single-blind or double-blind test administered in the office, in which the allergen is incorporated into "safe" food, where it will be hidden from the patient's view, paired with a purely "safe" food—to test for a placebo effect—and then the patient is monitored for a response.

Many doctors question the efficacy of such a formal testing route. Single-blind testing is useful only if the doctor is a good actor whose body language and lines of questioning won't tip the patient off to which bite contains the allergen. Allergists are not used to having to fool their patients, especially young ones. Double-blind testing requires the intervention of a third party to create food samples, and the prep work and subsequent monitoring can stretch each test into a six-hour session. This isn't realistic for the schedule of a lot of families, and it's a financial loss for the doctors. Most HMOs equate testing to a single "appointment," no matter how long it takes, and compensate accordingly.

So most families end up testing at home, one lick and nibble and half spoonful at a time. Once, I was telling someone about the process when, unfamiliar with the terms I was using, he stopped me and asked, " 'Food challenge?' As in, Sandra versus peanut?"

Kind of. Though I've always thought of it more in terms of Russian roulette.

CHAPTER TWO

Surviving Childhood

Raising you," my mother has said more than once, "was a full-time job." Soon after my diagnosis of multiple food allergies, the doctors charged her with narrowing down the list of specific culprits. My mother, the lab scientist. This is the first of many ad hoc professions forced upon the parent of a child with allergies.

When I was five months old, she followed orders by giving me a small, exploratory lick of an ice cream cone. Not many children holler *after* getting their ice cream. She could hear my cries hoarsening by the second as my throat began to swell. She added that noise to the dictionary of cries developed by all new moms: hungry cry, attention-hungry cry, overtired cry, scared cry, and now closing-airway cry.

The rest of my reaction vocabulary slowly emerged. Often I

tried to ignore an attack at first, embarrassed I might have done something wrong and fearing the trouble that would follow. The giveaway was the audible wheezing as my asthma kicked in. I made a peculiar *squonk* sound when the back of my mouth itched: a loud, convulsive flexing of tongue against palate that I still do today, often four or five times in a row, unaware I'm even doing it. My mother took to watching for these warning flares, sometimes recognizing a reaction before I had fully admitted it to myself.

One night, when I was ten, she secretly switched from using hard-to-find Fleischmann's sunflower margarine (unsalted sticks only—not regular, not "light," not in the tub) to a new, more widely available nondairy spread. She was tired of having to hunt through three different grocery stores every time she went shopping. I noticed the mashed potatoes were a little smoother and more golden but figured it had to do with using russets versus Yukon Golds. After my first few bites, I noticed her watching me. Intently. "Do you like the mashed potatoes?" she asked.

"Yeah," I said. "Why?"

"Well, you're rubbing at your mouth like you do sometimes when your lips itch." (My mother, the detective.)

One round of *squonk*ing and a Benadryl later, I was sleeping it off and she was tossing the impostor spread in the trash. The next day she got out her shopping list. *Fleischmann's*, she added back. *Unsalted*.

When a reaction struck my esophageal system, I could describe the inflammation only in terms of "bubbles" rising up in my chest. The frequency and intensity of the pressure, which seemed to rise, swell, and pop in waves, then had to be converted into usable medical information on whether the Benadryl was working. "This is serious," I remember my mother saying in frustration while on the phone with a Kaiser Permanente nurse. "She says the bubbles are getting bigger."

There were always concerned phone calls—if not to our HMO then to her father or brother, both doctors. My grandfather was a navy officer who had worked with NASA's space program. He was used to treating stoics and was initially skeptical about the severity of my allergies. On one of my first visits to my grandparents' house, I scooped my finger into a bowl of cottage cheese and then touched my cheek. Within seconds, a line of hives rose up. That was when he became a believer.

We were fortunate to never encounter disbelievers among the staff and teachers at my schools. Or their skepticism, if present, was trumped by their fear of lawsuits. They wanted to help—assuming we could just, please, get those forms turned in first. Please. In duplicate. Every year brought one form for my Benadryl, one for my inhaler, one for my EpiPen; one note for field trips, one for allergy shots, and one requesting the early lunch shift, when the cafeteria tables were cleanest. Every year, slightly different versions required precise wording and fresh signatures. (My mother, the contracts lawyer.)

Once I was in school, my mother went from being the one making the calls to the one who received them. Constantly. Even after you create a protocol for lunch, food pops up in a myriad of settings. When we read Dr. Seuss in second-grade story time, the class made green eggs and ham. In art class, we used pasta shells and wheels for texture. We were studying the Spanish explorers in world history, so was there a kind of taco I could eat? Could I try the funnel cake on Field Day?

Rather than try to shepherd from afar, my mother simply came along on field trips. Accidents still happened. When thirty kids from our elementary school went to the Benihana Japanese steakhouse for lunch, I ran over to my mom to share my news: "I can eat steak!"

"How do you know that?" she asked.

"I just ate some! A bite. Can I have more?"

In the chaos of a hibachi table, I had been diced a portion of teriyaki beef instead of chicken. I not only lived to tell the tale, but for a honeymoon period I could eat steak. My mom, sensing that it was a fluke, restricted access to either very special home-cooked meals or when absolutely nothing else was available, and never more than a small portion. Even with only infrequent exposure, my mast cells soon caught on to the cow. The reactions began, and became quite vicious quite quickly. My farewell bite of filet mignon was in 1991, followed by an hour of making *squonk*ing noises as I curled up on the couch.

Given my spectrum of issues—a variety of allergens, a capacity for anaphylaxis, and an ability to develop new sensitivities upon repeated exposure—my allergies constitute a disability. I am protected under the Rehabilitation Act of 1973, Section 504, and the Americans with Disabilities Act of 1990. Had my parents judged a school ineffective in managing my food allergies, they would have had legal recourse to insist on a binding "504 Plan," including an individual health plan (IHP) that would have covered everything from evaluating my capacity for self-care to listing all my allergies and their attack symptoms to naming safe food substitutions. They could have demanded that a "Severe Food Allergy Alert" flyer be posted throughout the school. They could have confirmed that my bus driver (by name) had been instructed not to allow eating on the ride to school.

In other words, they could have swatted a fly with a machete. But for every forty times a 504 Plan would be overkill, there might be the one time when it is critical. Back when I was a kid, and food was being handed out to everyone else, my "accommodation" equaled having the teachers know not to give me a share. True accommodation would have been providing a comparable substitute, but I was too embarrassed to ask.

That said, what if the food being given to me had been my main food for the day? I remember one kid in the class who lived off those snacks, because he didn't get anything at home. For students receiving free or reduced-rate meals, it's hard enough accepting help without being made to feel like Oliver Twist, pleading for more gruel because it is the only edible thing on your plate. A 504 Plan provides outside leverage.

But it takes a lot of red tape to weave together a safety net. A typical IHP consists of sections A through O that include a list of participating parties, doctor's letters, a narrative summary, and fine print. The plan can antagonize school officials by priming them to worry about liability. For most kids, an emergency action plan (EAP) will do—a less formal but still informative document that focuses on crisis moments. The most common one uses a format endorsed by the Food Allergy and Anaphylaxis Network (FAAN) and can be downloaded for free from their website.

One day, years out of school and visiting my mother's house for coffee, I showed her a copy of an EAP. It included a square for the child's photo and a checkbox for reaction-exacerbating asthma. Step one described "Treatment," a range of symptoms matched to a checkable set of options to give epinephrine or antihistamine, with additional space to note the dosages. "Step 2: Emergency Calls" provided a field for a doctor and a field for a parent, with the addendum "Do not hesitate to medicate or take child to a medical facility!" The form offered a place to identify three school staff members trained at using EpiPens or Twinjects, and—in case none of the staff could be located—illustrated instructions on how to administer the injection.

My mother took in the generously sized blanks, the bold-face type, the arrows showing which end of the EpiPen to pull off when activating it. She shook her head.

"Yeah, this is all new," she said. "This would have been nice."

A primary motivator for these standardized plans was a 1992 study on fatal and near-fatal food-induced anaphylaxis in children and teens, in which it was shown that four out of the six deadly attacks (but none of the seven near fatalities) recorded in the study took place in school. In other words, allergic children are offered some protection from potentially fatal allergens by the bulwark of a school environment. But once exposure *has* occurred, the bureaucracy of classroom decision-making (to give Benadryl, or EpiPen? one Benadryl, or two? does the teacher administer the EpiPen, or should the school nurse?) can cost precious minutes and therefore lives. And in fact, all the in-school fatalities were associated with appreciable delays of epinephrine injection. The minimum delay was twenty minutes. On average, seventy-five minutes usually elapsed before an injection occurred.

In Ontario, Canada, the death of thirteen-year-old Sabrina Shannon, who had an allergic reaction to curds on cafeteria French fries and subsequently collapsed in the hall of her high school, was partially attributable to a delay in epinephrine treatment. Her mother, Sara Shannon, became a crusader for laws requiring fixed anaphylactic response plans in schools. This sparked a piece of legislation known as "Sabrina's Law," and a wrenching documentary by the same name.

Granted, every child with potential for anaphylaxis should carry epinephrine within immediate reach and be trained to instruct those around them on when and how to use it. But younger kids might not be able to grasp the concept—or might forget all their lessons when panicked for breath. Worse yet, some anaphylactic reactions (as many as 19 percent, according to one study) require two injections before the emergency crews even arrive. Given that an insurance-covered EpiPen costs fifty dollars a pop, and the dose has only a year-long shelf life, to ask every child to carry two is a significant financial burden. There should be an unexpired epinephrine injector in every school's first aid kit, in a known and unlocked location, that can be used to augment an allergic child's primary supply.

If there's one thing becoming more and more obvious, it's that teachers need the means and the permission to pull the trigger on epinephrine. I know that's scary. An injection necessitates a trip to the emergency room, whereas the alternate plan is to let the Benadryl-dosed child (who will protest violently that she is *fine*, as she puffs on her inhaler) sleep it off in the clinic. But the side effects of an EpiPen's worth of epinephrine are usually no worse than tremor, nausea, and a mild headache. The side effect of anaphylaxis is death.

Even my mother, with all of her experience, sighs over the countless times she should have used my EpiPen and did not.

"You were so lucky," she says. "We were so lucky."

• • •

By the time I got to high school, I had become increasingly aware of foods that made no conceptual sense. Cheesecake, for example. Cake should not be cheesy. Cheese should not be caked. Admittedly, I had never tasted cheese. Nor had I ever eaten anything like the spongy, frosting-rich, boxed-mix-plus-egg cakes that populated the parties of my friends. But curdled milk served at room temperature? With cherries on top? This is what dessert would look like on the island of Doctor Moreau.

So when I found myself being herded with a crowd of friends into a restaurant known for its all-cheesecake menu, I knew I was in trouble. We were on a choir trip to New York, where we were booked to sing at Carnegie Hall. My mother's instructions echoed in my head: *Watch for pickpockets. Don't walk over sidewalk grates in a skirt. Keep those medicines on you at all times.*

She should have added *Avoid restaurants with a fifteen-dollar-per-person minimum.* There wasn't a single menu item I could eat. I asked for a root beer.

"A root beer float, you mean," the waiter said.

"No, I can't have ice cream. Can I just get a root beer? And what brand is it?"

"A and W."

"Oh." I was pretty sure A&W's recipe included egg whites, to make the head frothier. "Just a Coke, then."

The waiter glared at me over his notepad. "That's not enough."

"Lay off her," Liz said. "Everyone else is ordering."

"Jeez, mister," someone else muttered. "You'll get your money."

We had the swagger of fifteen-year-olds out on the town. At the Empire State Building, a junior-year tenor had announced that an object dropped from the Observation Deck would gain so much momentum that if it hit a person walking below, it would punch into his skull. We'd pitched our pennies anyway, little Lincoln bombs plummeting toward the sidewalk. We were renegades.

After taking the other ten orders, the waiter jabbed his Bic pen behind his ear and stalked off. I scuffed my shoes back and forth against the checkerboard linoleum. I was the only one who had already changed into the prescribed stage costume of a white button-down shirt, black skirt, and black tights. My purse was stuffed with an EpiPen, an inhaler, Kleenex, and six Benadryl. I had chosen the black purse, hoping the conductor wouldn't notice it onstage. The odds of a Parmesan ambush at Carnegie Hall were low, but I'd promised my mother.

The waiter came back with ten plates, ten forks, and one Coke with watery ice. When he slammed my glass down, soda slopped onto the table.

"Can I have a napkin?" I asked.

"Get one from your friends," he said, turning away. "Only plates come out with napkins."

Once he was gone, my friends fumed at his rudeness. Someone suggested we dine and dash. Someone suggested we talk to the manager. Drunk with power and engorged on cheese-cake, my friends decided his punishment: they would stiff him on the tip.

By now it was six o'clock, and we were due back at the hotel in our stage outfits. The two Jens put their money down. "Gotta run and change." One girl had to go meet her mother, who was chaperoning. The three altos sharing a room headed out. Then the other sopranos followed them. I was the last one at the table.

Our waiter swooped down on the pile of cash. He eyed me, counting out each bill.

"Where's my tip?"

"Um..." I froze. "I don't think they wanted to give you one."

With a loud clatter he swept ten dirty plates into a plastic dish tub. Then he picked up the tub and stormed through the double-hinged doors, cursing in an unidentifiable language. From the kitchen I heard the crash of the tub being thrown to the floor. Only then did I do what I should have done ten minutes before: I ran.

I had always been a careful, obedient child, figuring that my allergies didn't give me much of a choice. In high school, I was ready to rebel. Teenage rebellion usually involves a sip of beer or a surreptitious make-out session during *Days of Thunder.* My coup took the form of a spoonful of peas.

I was sitting on the far left end of the L-shaped sectional that anchored our downstairs. For years my regular seat had been the prime real estate on the far right end of the couch. Bigger end table. Close to the window. But my kid sister's macaroni-and-cheese habit had contaminated that section of furniture; the ghosts of countless fumbled pasta bears past haunted the armrest, residual dairy causing my eyes to water whenever I sat there. I had been forced to relocate.

"I've spent years facing the TV from a different angle," I whined to my mom. "Now my neck feels strained."

Dinner that night was one of the usual combinations of baked chicken breast, wild rice, and boiled peas. No sauces, no garnishes, Sandra-friendly. As I lifted the obligatory vegetable to my mouth, it occurred to me that I didn't particularly like peas.

In fact, I hated peas.

I could hate peas!

It was the first time I could remember articulating a dislike of something I'd eaten. I'd grown up thinking of food in terms of two categories—deadly and safe. I had a few favorites, sure (bacon, French fries, artichokes in chicken broth). But outright "dislikes" were a luxury only others could afford.

On the secure shores of my family's tan shag carpet, I decided I deserved to have dislikes like anyone else. The moratorium on peas would last seven years. Later in life, I'd take to turning down okra, *uni*, Israeli couscous, and red onions. I admit that cavalierly saying no to something on a menu still thrills me a little.

If only all my problems could have been solved by swapping peas for lima beans. In the course of three years, I had gone from being a cute, eager-to-please kid to being a moody lump of greasy hair and sweaty armpits. I rolled my jean shorts up so high that the pocket linings showed. I chewed gum just so I could snap it in sullen comment.

Fifteen was the year we discontinued my allergy shots, after a new round of testing revealed they'd had little impact on my sensitivities. Just what every teenager craves: incontrovertible evidence that she's been duped by The Man.

"Fourteen goddamn years of goddamn injections and they didn't do a goddamn thing," I reported to my friends. Actually, the shots probably kept my environmental allergies from worsening, but such subtleties were lost on me. I had just discovered cynicism, which required modifying sentences with "goddamn" whenever possible.

I turned rude toward any and all doctors. I "forgot" to use my daily inhalers. When chided, I muttered, "It's my body."

My mother would pick me up for dentist appointments and ask if I'd brushed my teeth. The answer was always a principled "No." I figured that if the dentist really needed to know what my teeth looked like, he should see them in their natural state. No playing nice with Crest and Scope.

I was insufferable. I was a teenager.

Life-or-death decisions fall into the hands of a food-allergic adolescent. As when you hand your Volvo keys over to a sixteen-year-old, it's invariable that accidents, even tragedies, are going to happen. A survey of one registry of food-induced anaphylaxis indicated that 69 percent of fatalities in a given year were victims between the ages of thirteen and twenty-one.

Say a teenager is heading out for a basketball game. He's wearing mesh shorts and a T-shirt, with his wallet and keys on a chain. He figures, *Where would I keep an EpiPen? Besides, I won't be eating anyway.* Then the players get swept along to a postgame pizza party. He's starved for carbs and surrounded by his buddies, and he doesn't want to be the weird guy asking if someone made absolutely sure there are no anchovies on the pie. So he thinks, *To hell with it, I've had pizza before.* He takes a bite.

In one study sponsored by the Food Allergy and Anaphylaxis Network, 54 percent of a pool of teenagers with severe allergies indicated purposefully ingesting a food known to contain at least a tiny amount of an allergen. Nearly half of those kids cited the rationale "It looked good and I wanted to eat it."

Most parents know to expect Superman Syndrome from their kids. According to that study, the good news is that teenagers with allergies, unlike most, know they're vulnerable. The bad news is, many don't care—at least, not enough to sit at the peanut-free lunch table or teach their friends how to use an EpiPen or wear jeans with pockets roomy enough for an inhaler. In an earlier study, the same team of doctors found that teenagers said that the hardest part of living with food allergies was "social isolation." Their parents cited the most difficult issue as "fear of death."

I was worried about both. I rolled my eyes when my mother suggested that I wear a MedicAlert bracelet ("They've gotten much more fashionable!"). But underneath the surliness, I couldn't shake that nutritionist's curse from years earlier. I was tired of eating baked chicken and boiled vegetables, tired of having to be careful all the time, tired of being broken. Shots hadn't fixed me. Was I unfixable? Was I unfit to survive?

This was the mid-1990s. It would be another ten years before a team of American psychologists ran a series of experiments on the neuropsychiatric effects of allergy, with grant support from the National Institute of Mental Health, NARSAD, and the American Foundation for Suicide Prevention. The scientists induced allergies to pollen and chicken egg in rats and mice. The test subjects were placed in an "open arena," akin to releasing a human onto an empty basketball court, and their motions were tracked. With controls in place for physical activity, an animal's confidence was measured by its willingness to venture into the center space. The allergy-ridden subjects chose to run along the walls of the arena, while normal creatures ventured out into the open.

"Little Mouse" had been one teacher's nickname for me in middle school, after she'd noticed I always ate bread from the inside out, nibbling my way around potentially egg-brushed crusts. The little mouse had grown into a teenager with an over-developed sense of mortality. I was an anxious creature, clinging to the walls of my arena.

High-strung teenagers are no more rare than rebellious ones. But the X factor of my adolescence, the ingredient that threatened to turn the cocktail toxic, was Benadryl. Benadryl was my ostensible savior—the one thing that could stave off a reaction without requiring a trip to the hospital—and so we had it stashed everywhere. At least six pills in my purse; in my mother's purse; in my locker; in the glove compartment of the car.

The maximum safe dosage of Benadryl within a given day is 300 milligrams. More than that can trigger ringing in the ears, dilated pupils, flushing, fever, hallucinations, and seizure. The bright, friendly shade of pink associated with the brand belies its powerful effects. If you've taken one, you should not be driving. Diphenhydramine, after all, is not just the active ingredient in Benadryl. Known for inducing drowsiness, it is the active ingredient in sleeping aids like Nytol, Unisom gels, and Tylenol PM.

Imagine a depressed housewife who is trying to shut out the siren call of sleeping pills. Now imagine she finds sleeping pills tucked in every pocket, every corner of the house, and even the penny dish by the front door. Imagine her husband reminding her before she leaves for the library or the movies or the grocery store: "Hey, do you have your sleeping pills with you? Do you need extra? Maybe you should pack a few extra."

Sometimes my friends would joke that if we ever decided to kill ourselves, I had the tastiest options by far. "Death by chocolate!" they exclaimed. "Death by ice cream!" It certainly would be easy. I can walk into any typical kitchen and find at least fifteen things that would kill me if I ate them, and that's without even looking under the sink for the drain cleaner.

Yet to anyone who has ever had a severe allergic reaction—the numb lips, the swollen throat, the frantic swallowing for air, the churning cramps—the idea that you would volunteer for that sensation is idiotic. Forget the allure of something sugary. No one wants to be drowning in their own spit as they die.

Benadryl was different. I knew what it tasted like (nothing at all), how easily one went down, how quickly another four or five could go down, how it made my eyelids sweetly heavy within a half hour. To an anxious and sleep-starved teenager attending a high-pressure high school, that didn't sound like such a bad way to go. At times that sounded like heaven.

One night I was hiding out in my room, moping and listening to Nirvana's *MTV Unplugged*. My parents were fighting. A boy I liked didn't like me back. I had a ten-page paper due the next day that I had not even started. I emptied my purse, rooted through my underwear drawer, reached into the sliding cubby of my headboard, unpeeled each individual blister casing, and lined up every capsule I had: fourteen Benadryl, and I hadn't even raided the upstairs. I looked at them for a long time. Then I burst into tears, hit the stop button on my boom box, and walked out to the living room. My mother, inured to the teenage temperament at this point, didn't ask questions. We sat on the couch together and watched the eleven o'clock news.

I used to wonder if I was the only one tempted to overdose. As I grew older and began meeting other people with allergies, we would crack wise on our membership in the cult of Benadryl carriers. There is no diplomatic way of asking, "So, did you ever think about taking a whole handful at once?"

Only as the world has become Googlable do I find them out there: The high school basketball player who died with a mixture of Benadryl and rubbing alcohol in his stomach. A paper on "pediatric intravenous catheter abuse," published after a child with long-term illness drained the powder from Benadryl capsules into her IV. And I wonder how many other kids, afraid they will always be at odds with the rest of the world, take a Benadryl or maybe two or maybe three—only to have nothing worse come of it than cotton mouth and a hellishly difficult time getting up for school the next morning.

That night, my mom went to bed after the news, but I stayed up to watch the *Tonight Show*. After the *Tonight Show* I watched the *Late Show*. Then the even later show. Then an infomercial starring Cher. Finally the station showed the American flag waving, while playing a prerecorded version of "The Star-Spangled Banner," followed by the blare of off-air static. By then I could barely keep my eyes open. I returned to my room and crawled straight under the covers. The pills, which I'd lined up along the foot of my moon-and-stars bedspread, scattered onto the floor.

. . .

When I was younger, eating outside the house was a family affair. My mother knew my allergies better than I did, so she did the ordering. No matter how careful we were, there were dozens of evenings derailed by attacks: my mother breaking out the Benadryl, my father interrogating the chef, and—if pills didn't work—driving to a hospital where we could hang out in the ER lobby until my airway opened up again.

"Just breathe," my father told me on one outing as I curled up in his lap, apologizing over and over for wasting our tickets to an art exhibit, a trip we had planned for weeks with my grandparents. "Calm down. Just breathe."

Even in high school, when friends took to dinner-and-movie nights, I stayed wedded to the three-person unit that managed what I ate and took care of me when something went wrong. In my parents' absence I might order French fries, and there was one—one—Japanese restaurant near school where I could trust the vegetable and chicken tempura. But that was it. Nothing else was worth the risk.

You can't make it through college on four years of potatoes. So before I took up residence on the grounds of the University of Virginia, my parents arranged a meeting with a supervisor who shared the entire index of the recipes used in UVA's cafeterias. "We'll take care of her," she promised.

The reality was less promising. I'd venture to the dining hall and watch servers use tongs to pass out corn bread, then use those same tongs to serve me an ear of corn. I'd look down at a plate now contaminated with buttermilk crumbs, shake my head, get a new plate, and start again. Theoretically, the university had pledged to my parents that Aramark would have a "safe protein" available at every dinner shift. The "safe protein" in question turned out to be completely unseasoned cod. Two slabs. Every time.

Part of the problem was that the dining hall was open for three-hour stretches; neither the staff nor I knew when I would arrive from day to day. Sometimes no one had remembered to defrost the fish and fire the plate, meaning a twenty-minute wait before it could be ready (an eternity in college time). More often the dish had been nuked, cling-wrapped, and stashed under a heat lamp at least an hour before I arrived. As I peeled off the covering, a stream of fishy, lukewarm condensation would run onto my plastic tray. The flesh would be rubbery to the touch.

"My god," someone at the table would say. "What is that?"

The day that broke me was when I walked in to hear a man in a plastic hairnet call back into the kitchen, "Yo, the fish girl's here!"

I took to dishing up white rice instead, ladled with chickpeas from the salad bar. But that worked only if I got to the salad bar before other students had contaminated the bins with drips of ranch dressing, which always seemed to slop out of the ladle as it was poured, or shreds of cheddar cheese. When that happened, my refuge was a bowl of dry Corn Pops. I had to suck on them before chewing so they didn't scrape the roof of my mouth. My allergies took one of dorm life's great culinary gifts—breakfast for dinner—and rendered it punitive.

Facing these culinary disasters, I couldn't resist taking a chance on the recipe du jour from time to time, asking first if it was Sandra-friendly. My first semester at school, on the first weekend my long-distance boyfriend came to visit, I was trying to impress him with how well I'd acclimated to being away from home. When he said the risotto looked good, I asked the server if it had any dairy in it. She assured me it didn't. I got a heaping plateful.

"They take good care of me here," I bragged. I don't know why I thought eating risotto would impress him. Maybe I was just afraid he wouldn't kiss me if I had cod breath. If I'd known the very definition of risotto stipulates cheese stirred into the rice as it cooks, I wouldn't have touched it. But I'd never heard of risotto. It looked like vegetables in rice, not that different from what I assembled myself via the salad bar.

My tongue told another story. On the first bite, strands of cheese (which I realized was what I had seen stretching from rice to fork) formed a strychnine web across the back of my throat. I took a long sip of water, continuing my serene chatter about classes as I assessed the damage. My boyfriend knew better than to believe my calm.

"Sandra?" he asked. "You okay?"

This was how I learned that an ambulance squad can reach any building on UVA's grounds in ten minutes, using paved shortcuts specifically designed for quick access. They came in with a wheelchair. Though my vision was blurring, and I felt woozy, I refused. I was not going to be seen being carted out of Newcomb Hall.

"Just use the chair," my boyfriend pleaded. But instead I marched out of the dining hall on my own feet, with my boyfriend and a four-person EMS crew behind me.

"Slow down!" said the tech wheeling the chair.

No way. I was hoping that if I walked fast enough, people would not realize they were there with me. In my mind, this was like some slow-motion Scorsese chase scene. Odds are that the tech was no more than a foot behind me, poised to catch me in case I collapsed backward.

The sequence that followed was one that would become familiar in the four years to come: Landing in the waiting room of the University of Virginia hospital, with its drooping potted palms and out-of-date copies of *Sports Illustrated.* Getting a dirty look from the father of a six-year-old with a broken arm, who had been waiting for an hour, while I went straight in—potential anaphylaxis goes to the top of the triage list. Refusing an IV, because I dread the bruise, followed by a lecture on refusing IVs. Benadryl, Zyrtec, and hours of lonely, bored, not-allowed-to-fall-asleep waiting on an ER cot while my boyfriend, equally lonely and bored, waited in the lobby. A man on the other side of the curtain kept whimpering about his leg.

The next time I went to the dining hall, they put out the plate of fish before I even had a chance to ask.

I sometimes took the bus to Harris Teeter for groceries. But I had nowhere to keep food, nowhere to cook it, and no money to spend. Besides, for the first time in my life, staying in to eat was no protection from the reach of dairy. My roommate was a nice Montana girl who liked pizza. Sometimes she'd talk on the phone while eating a slice. If I used the same phone to make a call, even hours later, oil left on the receiver raised hives all along my chin and cheek.

This led to an awkward lecture about keeping surfaces clean. In every dorm, someone gets stuck with the lame roommate assignment. Once you have uttered the phrase "baby wipes" to another eighteen-year-old, face it: you are that lame roommate.

Whenever my mother heard about these reactions, she was furious on my behalf. One morning, I explained I had missed her phone call the night before because I'd been inadvertently exiled from our suite, when my roommate popped buttered popcorn in the microwave next to my bed. She told me to be more assertive. "This is a matter of life and death," she said. "They have to understand that."

But I wanted so badly to be something other than the fussy one. Four years of college and countless reactions never quashed the dream that I could be just another UVA 'Hoo, in all her sloppy glory.

At a postgraduation beach week, my drunken housemates decided to turn beer pong into "White Russian pong," sending a spray of milk and Kahlúa into the air every time someone plunked a Ping-Pong ball into a Solo cup. I didn't object. I stood by, cheering for a team, not touching anything, hoping for the best.

After an hour, so much milk had been splashed about that I started to react. On autopilot, I ordered my boyfriend to drive to a nearby ER, where I hung out in the lobby, waiting for the Benadryl to work. He settled in and watched cable TV. I lay down on a scratchy couch nearby, stared at the ceiling, and tried to relax.

I didn't fit in anyone's lap anymore. No one knew to say "Breathe. Just breathe." The protective bubble of life with my family had burst, and I was on my own.

CHAPTER THREE

Eat, Drink, and Be Wary

Rituals mark every life. Traditions and celebrations affirm membership in a group or provide comfort in daily repetition or declare passage from one stage to the next. Yet the reality is that my eighteenth birthday party didn't make me an adult. Nor did graduating from college. Even when I moved into my first postcollege apartment, with my dad as a cosigner on the lease, I felt like a kid playing dress-up.

But learning that my best friend Kristen was getting married finally dropped the anvil of adulthood on my head. Not just a best friend but *the* best friend—the one I'd had for ten years, who'd watched me cry over my high school sweetheart; the one with whom I shared an invented code consisting of the words *bob, funk, derf,* and, on special occasions, *pampelmousse.* How had the volunteer fireman our friends had teased Kristen about transmogrified into the future father of her children? Where did that leave me?

That left me in a booth of St. Maarten Café, celebrating to the tune of "Another One Bites the Dust." Four of us had gathered on a Friday night in Charlottesville, Virginia, on the Corner, the strip of bars we had frequented back as UVA undergrads. Not too froufrou, not too grimy, Maarten's—as the students call it—is the kind of tavern where regular visits earn you a mug with your name inscribed on the bottom. Kristen liked to order the bananas Foster, complete with flaming ice cream. Eric and Dave preferred the loaded waffle fries, buried under a layer of melted cheese. I planned to do my part by getting a round of shots for all.

While they deliberated about the food, I scrutinized the laminated place mat that doubled as a drink menu, looking for something Sandra-friendly that didn't contain Irish cream, Midori, or chocolate. The house specialties cater to someone who has the sweet tooth of a five-year-old and the sense of humor of a fifteen-year-old. No other explanation justifies the Buttery Nipple.

"What about Lemon Drops?" I asked my friends. Vodka, with a sugar-rimmed glass and a wedge of lemon afterward. Sweet, simple, and wickedly effective. My parents had not raised a lightweight. As my mother had once said, "We're just glad you can enjoy *something* fun."

When the waitress brought out a quartet of shot glasses, the vodka looked a little cloudy. But some bartenders add a squeeze of lemon, and I wasn't going to make everyone wait while I asked questions. Rail vodka is drinkable only as long as it is ice cold, and already our fingertips were melting away the frost on each small glass.

"To Kristen and Fireman Bob!" we toasted.

The next day I would call the bar and learn that what I had ordered was not a round of Lemon Drops but a round of St. Maarten's Signature Lemon-Drop Shooters, in which the vodka is accented with a dash of sour mix. Commercial drink mixes, as any student of chemistry or cheap margaritas might tell you, contain a boatload of ingredients that separate rather unappealingly over time. So a milk derivative is added as a binder. It may be way down there, fifteenth or sixteenth in the small print of ingredients, but it's there.

In that moment in Maarten's, I knew none of this. What I knew, as soon as I set my drained shot glass back on the table, was that my esophagus was on fire. What on earth? Vodka, lemon, sugar: I wasn't allergic to any of those things. What was I missing? Had the glass been dirty from someone else's Buttery Nipple?

This cannot happen, I thought. This was Kristen's night, and the point of coming to Charlottesville was to show that I was excited for her. It would not be an auspicious gesture to toast her new life, then vomit.

I tried to be nonchalant as I excused myself to go to the restroom, a two-stalled cave that smelled like a bachelor party. Making a bad situation worse was the fact that unlike with a typical reaction, I had not stopped after a trial bite. I was at the mercy of the full shot, my entire throat coated. After a few minutes, I staggered out to our table.

"Um, guys," I said. "I'm gonna need your help."

The night was supposed to be my treat, but someone else must have paid the bill while I waited outside, head resting against my knees. We walked what seemed like an eternal four blocks back to Dave's apartment. I refused Eric's offer to carry me. I refused to go to the hospital, hoping two Benadryl would be enough.

"Damn it," I said, stumped, "I didn't even *eat* anything."

When we got inside, I dashed to the bathroom. My friends watched TV on the couch and took turns coming to check on me. I had started the night with a shot, and I ended it curled up around Dave's toilet, worshipping the feel of the cool tile against my skin. A quintessential night of college drinking, minus much actual drinking.

If I'd been by myself, I would have said, "Can you check with the bartender on the ingredients?" Or I would have taken a test sip, then waited a few minutes. But this was not a drink; this was a toast. To question or hesitate violates the ritual. It's like going to a dinner party and salting your host's dish before the first taste. It's a matter of trust.

Rituals trump our usual food inhibitions. Oktoberfest? Sure, I'll cool myself off with a full pitcher of Hefeweizen. County fair? Bring on the deep-fried Oreos. Seafood feast? Why, yes, slurping three-dozen oysters in ten minutes *does* sound like a good idea. This is what happens when you cross rites of consumption with mob mentality.

Some foods carry such heft of tradition that their preparation or serving becomes the focus of the day. Spaghetti Mondays. Chili cook-offs. Domino's delivery. Even my parents, on some nights when they rented a movie to watch, couldn't resist ordering in pizza. I was given the sacred duty of sprinkling the red chili pepper, performing this rite with an enthusiasm that must have scorched the roofs of their mouths.

Eventually, my mother gave in to my begging and fixed me my own faux "pizza": salt-and-water dough that couldn't raise a proper crust, layered in tomato sauce straight out of a can and a few sautéed onions. We grimaced our way through three slices. It was bad, but not quite so bad as when I would run hot water out of the kitchen tap, dump in salt and pepper, and sit by the fireplace to eat my "soup." Sure, my mother sometimes made broth, but I wanted to be like those kids in the Campbell's soup ads. I wanted to pretend I was having cream-of-whatever, complete with all-natural flavors, hydrolyzed proteins, and whatever it was that equaled "tasty" for everyone else and "deadly" for me. I never made it past a couple of spoonfuls before admitting that this was nothing like what I'd seen in the commercials.

All the rites of eating I've ever envied have been secular—defined by pop culture, geography, or my era. But in scenarios where the ritual is religious, and strictly codified, those with food allergies or other dietary restrictions experience a more profound exclusion. Around 2001, a controversy arose when Boston's Roman Catholic Church (seconded by the Archdiocese of New York) affirmed its decree that rice-based wafers were not an acceptable substitute for wheat-based Communion wafers—even for those unable to ingest wheat.

The Communion tradition is grounded in the story of the Last Supper, at which Jesus ate unleavened wheat bread and shared wine with his disciples. This meal is re-created during Sunday services, when Catholics accept into their mouths bread that has been consecrated as the body of the Savior, as well as a sip of wine that embodies His blood. Eastern

Orthodox churches typically use unfermented grape juice and cubes of leavened bread cut from a *prosphorá* loaf, referred to as the Eucharist. Westernized Christianity, including Roman or Latin-rite Catholics, use unleavened wafers referred to as the host. The Church takes this transubstantiation very seriously—Martin Luther's questioning and ultimate denial of this principle was one of the primary catalysts of the Protestant Reformation. First Communion is a particularly elaborate ceremony, during which family and friends gather to watch as a child recites verses signifying an allegiance to God before accepting the host for the first time.

The Catholic Church's Code of Canon Law suggests that those who cannot tolerate the traditional host should opt for a "low-gluten wafer." The United States Conference of Catholic Bishops (USCCB) even goes so far as to recommend a specific supply, developed by the Benedictine Sisters of Perpetual Adoration in Clyde, Missouri, and endorsed by the magazine *Gluten-Free Living*, which can be mail-ordered from the Congregation's Altar Bread Department. When you consider the reaction I had to an infinitesimal fraction of "nonfat milk powder" in that shooter, it's hard to imagine even the lowest of low-gluten wafers feeling like an option for anyone with allergies or severe celiac disease. Throwing up the toast to my friend's engagement was a party foul; throwing up the body of our Savior would be straight out of *The Omen*.

For some Latin-rite Catholics, taking the wine (the Precious Blood) alone might carry its own complications. The chalice of wine, if communal, would be quickly contaminated by the mouths of everyone else who has taken the wheat-based host. The faithful might have an intolerance to alcohol. As a last resort, the Church states that a bishop may grant permission for someone to receive *mustum*, a wine with minimal alcohol content. If you can't take *mustum*, the Church shrugs its papal shoulders.

"There is little else the Church can do except to recommend that the person make a 'spiritual communion,'" says the FAQ answer issued by the USCCB's Committee on Divine Worship. "Why? Because the Church believes that it is impossible to consecrate anything except wheat bread and grape wine."

In many parishes, there is now leeway in the form of pastors who quietly supply nonwheat bread, wrapping the portions in foil to mark them as safe among the rest. But that's the exception, not the rule—and in fact, it is in explicit defiance of the rule. It's not as if the Vatican has turned a blind eye to the issue. In 1994, they issued a set of dictates for bishops that included this specific decree: "Special hosts [which do not contain gluten] are invalid matter for the celebration of the Eucharist." The author of this statement was the then cardinal Joseph Ratzinger, who has since ascended to become Pope Benedict XVI himself.

Or, as the pastor of Our Lady Help of Christians Parish was quoted as saying during a 2001 interview with the Associated Press at the time of the Boston controversy: "We many are sharing one bread and becoming one with Christ. We can't make different flavors for different folks and maintain that theological reality."

Explain that to those Catholic children affected by wheat allergy or celiac disease who have faithfully spent two years of Sunday school training with the other kids, when their studies lead up to getting their own little odd-man-out serving of wine and watching from the side as friends line up, hands cupped to receive the wafer.

Everyday practice concerning Communion has grown greatly more flexible in the last five years and will probably only continue to grow more accommodating. But there is still the issue, at the end of the day, of how the Church's chief philosophers have reconciled this "theological reality" with the post-Eden realm. Embedded in the Vatican policy seems to be the suggestion that allergies are a challenge to willpower rather than an absolute barrier; that those of true devotion could surely manage just one bite and one sip, just once a week. If the Church doesn't believe that, the alternative is what? That some of its followers are not biologically designed to be Catholic?

Some families, when confronted with their Church's resistance to their children's needs, respond by leaving the faith. The Catholic Church's loss is the gain of the Methodists, Episcopalians, and Evangelical Lutherans, who do not have such restrictive policies. The Lutheran Church says as much in section 44C of "The Use of the Means of Grace": "For pressing reasons of health . . . congregations might decide to place small amounts of non-wheat bread or non-alcoholic wine or grape juice on the altar. Such pastoral and congregational decisions are delicate, and must honor both the tradition of the Church and the people of each local assembly." For these forms of Christianity, the meaningful substance of Communion is in the symbolic presence of Jesus, not the grain used in the bread or the proof of the grape wine.

Perhaps it is crucial that the rite use the same recipe handed down for centuries, in an unbroken lineage, just as Latin phrasing is used to celebrate Mass long after the language has otherwise died out. I have never been Catholic. I can't judge. What I can do is speak to our own elementary-school sacrament: the birthday treat.

Every week without fail, it seemed, a different classmate would come to the front of the room and we would sing "Happy Birthday." We would sit at our desks as he or she walked down each row, arms wrapped around a large Tupperware container. One by one each child would raise upturned palms to receive a cupcake. When the birthday kid got to my seat, there would always be an awkward pause. That would remind the teacher to open the supplies cabinet, the same one that held the glitter and the paper towels, and pull out the bag of hazelnuts that my mother had dropped off on the first day of school that year.

Twelve hazelnuts. Precisely twelve hazelnuts would be counted out into my cupped hands. I'd line them up in the pencil groove at the top of my desk and ask if anyone else wanted one. No one else ever wanted one.

I'd try to match the pacing of everyone else's treat. Three hazelnuts as people licked off the frosting; three as people took huge bites of the moist, spongy cake; three as people licked the baking sleeves clean, scraping the last of the cake off with their teeth; and three final nuts that I would grind slowly into a paste that coated my back molars as the teacher went around the room with the wastebasket to collect wrappers and napkins.

When my birthday came, did I go around the room with a bag of hazelnuts and count out twelve to a kid? Of course not. I begged my mother to make cupcakes from the Duncan Hines mix, even though I wouldn't be able to eat one. The point wasn't what I could eat. The point was having my turn to walk around the room with that big box in my arms, the same as everyone else.

This was why I went trick-or-treating every year, knowing I'd have to give away everything but the lollipops, Life Savers, and raisins (I was probably the only child in Virginia who yelped in joy at being given raisins). This was why I sometimes taped Hershey's Kisses to my valentines, being careful to pick up only ones with perfectly intact foil wrapping. I wanted to fit in; I wanted to do it the same way everyone else did it. Any Catholic official surprised when a child is not satisfied by drinking the wine—while everyone else takes the host—has missed an essential point.

Is it inclusiveness that makes rituals valuable? Or is maintaining the ritual's integrity that matters, even if that leaves someone out? Maybe I should have glued boxes of raisins to my valentines, to make a point. But that's a slippery slope. Next thing you know, you're getting a *B Mine 4EVER* note taped to a roast chicken.

· · ·

There are many ways of ritualizing foods. Communion imbues otherwise modest substances with an air of mystery. In the secular world, we have our own way of elevating the everyday to the divine: the secret recipe.

"Good lord!" you exclaim, licking your fingers at dinner one night. "This is delicious. What's in this?"

"Oh, that's something my great-grandmother brought over from the old country," your hostess says. If you ask for the ingredients, she'll just lay a finger to her lips and shake her head in silence, smiling.

As a child I was embargoed from the world of secret ingredients. My mother approached the nutritional-information label of every box with a magnifying glass. My father pop-quizzed chefs on preparation techniques.

But then I went to the University of Virginia. If college is the bridge between childhood and adult life, perhaps it's fitting that it is home to many artificial secrets. We want to sit at the adult dinner table come Thanksgiving, yet we're not quite ready to give up the oath that gets us admission to the backyard tree house.

So we create clubs. We make up secrets for the sake of having secrets to keep. UVA had its plethora of secret societies including the Zs, the IMPs, the Seven Society, and the Society of the Purple Shadows. They give out student scholarships, paint emblems on the grounds, and lay wreaths on each anniversary of Mr. Jefferson's death, but their rosters are never divulged. The only acknowledgment of a Seven's identity is after his death, when the university chapel's bell is rung out seven times on the day of his burial.

I pledged the not-so-secret Jefferson Literary and Debating Society, whose history includes having had Woodrow Wilson as our president and Edgar Allan Poe as our secretary—not at the same time—and having sponsored one of the foundation stones of the Washington Monument. The "Jeff" has any number of rituals. Some have the briefest of heydays, such as the two years when a meeting could not be gaveled in until a Twinkie had been tossed up in the chandelier of the hall where we gathered on the Lawn's west range. One tradition that has endured is our official drink, the Whiskey Sour, which would be served at the five o'clock "Sippers," hosted by the Room Seven Resident before every Friday Society meeting.

The Sour recipe is handed down from one Room Seven Resident to another, and it is secret. Top secret. For my first few years of Society membership, I didn't ask about the recipe. But I was dying to stand around with everyone else sipping the official Society drink, rather than making do with Stingrays of Aristocrat gin and flat ginger ale. Going into my fourth year, a friend was named Room Seven Resident. I saw my chance.

"So, Eston. Any chance I could find out what's in the Whiskey Sours?"

"Nope."

I should have known that any student who was also an army reservist would be strict about following orders.

"Eston, I've gone three years without a Whiskey Sour."

"If I told you, I'd have to kill you."

Eventually we came to a compromise. Eston would send me a list that included the ingredients of the Whiskey Sours, as well as a number of red herrings. That way I could size up any potential dangers without actually learning the recipe. The list, when it arrived in my email, looked something like this:

Lime
Sprite
Spearmint
Worcestershire sauce
Cornstarch
7UP
Zima

Club soda
Orange juice
Cinnamon
Xanthan gum
Bitters
Sugar
Jalapeño
Grapefruit juice
Lemonade
Carbolic acid
Kosher salt
Basil
Fresca

There it was. Grapefruit juice. A few years earlier, I'd been on the road with my parents and, while going for orange juice at the continental breakfast bar, had accidentally poured a glass of grapefruit juice. One sip made me feel like a giant had reached into my chest, grabbed my heart, and squeezed tight. I dumped the glass out and took a deep draw on my inhaler. It might not have been a proper oral food challenge, but it was enough to make me avoid grapefruit from that day forward.

But did that mean I was allergic? At the time of that reaction, I was on Hismanal—a second-generation antihistamine that would later be pulled from the market when it was discovered it triggered potentially fatal interactions with CYP3A4 enzyme inhibitors, such as those found in . . . grapefruit juice.

With the Hismanal cleared from my system, knowing I didn't have any other citrus sensitivity, there was no reason not to try it again. That was the rational stance. And yet, knowing how it had made me feel that one time, I avoided it as carefully as any allergen. Once, a friend asked point-blank if I could have grapefruit.

"No," I said.

"So you're allergic?"

"Uh," I said. "Kinda. It gives me heart attacks."

Not only was grapefruit juice on the list, but it also seemed—unlike carbolic acid or Fresca—likely to be an actual ingredient. Perhaps it was time to try again. I pictured that first, hesitant sip. I pictured passing out on the floor of Room 7 West Lawn. No. Grapefruit would stay in limbo; I'd stick with my Stingrays. If I felt left out, I could try, extra hard, to be the one to lodge the Twinkie in the chandelier at 7:29 p.m. that Friday.

Though secret recipes will never be allergy friendly, I'm drawn to them—from the good (barbecue) to the gross (Tofutti). But their era, I suspect, is coming to an end.

Take Kentucky Fried Chicken. Eleven unknown herbs and spices, concocted by Colonel Sanders himself, supposedly give the chicken its unique flavor. What experience do I have with Kentucky Fried Chicken? The answer should be "none." In a perfect world my parents would never risk feeding me chicken dipped in a mystery mix, fried in who knows what oil, and dished in the same bag as butter-laced mashed potatoes.

But like most people, I am at the mercy of extended family. During visits to the sprawling horse farm in West Virginia once owned by my aunt and uncle, mealtime sometimes centered on buckets of KFC, which is a good quick fix when you've got five kids in the house. While everyone was grabbing pieces of chicken, I would assure my mom it was worth a shot.

She'd pick out a breast for me, the biggest she could find,

and make it Sandra-friendly. That meant peeling off the batter; then the creamy layer of fat swaddling the skin; then the top layer of the chicken itself. What remained—shreds of flesh clinging to bone—I happily accepted on my plate, like a baby robin taking regurgitated food from the mouth of her mama.

The idea for KFC goes all the way back to 1930, when Harland Sanders began serving fried chicken at a gas station he owned in Corbin, Kentucky. Sanders Court & Café earned a steady following, and in 1936, when Governor Ruby Laffoon stopped in for a bite, he rewarded the proprietor with the title of "Kentucky Colonel" in recognition of his mastery of the iron skillet.

Colonel Sanders was frying chicken by his own hand, which took about thirty minutes per piece. But as the operation grew—he annexed a nearby motel and turned it into a sit-down restaurant—he looked to streamline his operation. By 1939, he was using a pressure fryer, and by 1940, the secret Original Recipe was born. In 1952, the Colonel had acquired a co-owner from South Salt Lake, Utah, and the first Kentucky Fried Chicken outlet opened. Over the next decade, the franchise spread across the country.

Colonel Sanders left the company after a buyout in 1964. His disavowal of the KFC gravy, made in some exit interviews, was a key sign that his hold on the franchise's menu had weakened as its geographic reach had increased. Journalist George Ritzer described how Ray Kroc, the founder of McDonald's and Sanders's friend, remembered the Colonel declaring, "I had the greatest gravy in the world, and those sons of bitches—they dragged it out and extended it and watered it down. . . ."

Theoretically, his secret recipe endured. A single sheet of

yellowing paper recording ingredients and amounts, scribbled in the Colonel's own hand, was kept first in a filing cabinet with two combination locks, and later in a computerized vault. Company leaders claim that portions of the spice mix are assembled in several different locations around the country, to prevent the line workers from transcribing the complete process.

Ironically, the success of the Original Recipe is what has contributed to its downfall. As KFC became popular enough to open in more than eighty-five countries, they began modifying their core cuisine to suit wider audiences. They offer a "grilled" chicken option, in which the Original Recipe is treated as a spice rub, and an "extra-crispy" variation that double-dips in flour. I'm especially intrigued by the testing of a Famous Bowl, a modified shepherd's pie consisting of layers of mashed potatoes, gravy, corn, popcorn chicken, and cheese. The Famous Bowl would kill me at least four different ways. In India, the "hot and spicy" chicken flavor has proven more popular with the South Asian palate. In Taiwan, you can order a side of egg tarts or lotus root salad.

Moans can be heard emanating from the grave of Sanders, who died in 1980.

The integrity of the Colonel's secret recipe is gone for good, as is the ritual of its preparation. Some say that the nuance of his frying technique, which included a controlled shift in temperature after the first minute, cannot be replicated in the age of automatic deep fryers. Surely some of the flavor was lost when a class action lawsuit filed by Ralph Nader's Center for Science in the Public Interest (alleging that the use of partially hydrogenated cooking oils posed a flagrant and reckless threat to public health) forced KFC to switch to trans-fat-free soybean oil for use throughout the restaurant chain by April 2007.

In 1983, William Poundstone published *Big Secrets*, in which he set out to expose America's greatest "mysteries"—and assert, along the way, that many were nothing more than market-driven hoopla. He submitted an off-the-street sample of KFC for chemical analysis that revealed the batter's ingredient list to be no more complicated than flour, salt, black pepper, and MSG. MSG, monosodium glutamate, is the Chinese-food additive that enhances flavor and, people joke, makes you hungry for more within the half hour. Whatever the Original Recipe was, it has been traded in (at least at the street level, by managers of individual franchises) for cheap ingredients and simpler proportions.

Poundstone also publicized the secret ingredients of Coca-Cola Classic, which include vanilla extract, citrus oils, and lime juice. Part of me knows that if I had a lime allergy and could never figure out why Coca-Cola made my throat itch, I would be grateful to him. Yet when I picture Harland Sanders in his kitchen apron, adding a pinch of this, a pinch of that, I can't help but mourn the death of the secret-recipe ritual. The problem is, I am the problem. Those with food allergies are the patron saints of the fight against secret ingredients, and Congress has acted in our name.

. . .

As food sellers increased their investment in prepackaged products during the twentienth century, we lost the ability to run down the street and double-check whether the baker had brushed his breads with egg that morning. Bread went from having four to fourteen ingredients, including any number of chemical derivatives designed to increase its shelf life. The markers of a modern kitchen included the pull-tab soda, the TV dinner, and other containers designed to rob foods of their organic shape and provenance.

In Ralph Nader's introduction to *The Chemical Feast,* a 1970 critique of the Food and Drug Administration authored by regulatory affairs attorney Jim Turner, Nader issued a clarion call for transparency in the labeling of commercial foods. "Food is the most intimate consumer product," Nader observed. So why is it, he asked, that we know more about what goes into a can of dog food than about what goes into our own bellies?

By the mid-1970s, the FDA provided suggested guidelines for labels describing products in terms of basic nutritional values: protein, fats, carbohydrates, and so on. Some companies chose to obey these guidelines in response to an increasing popular interest in good health. After all, this was the beginning of the era of Richard Simmons (real name: Milton Teagle Simmons), whose rise to fitness guru fame was preceded by stints as a New Orleans pralines vendor, a New York advertising executive, and a Beverly Hills maître d'. Take that unholy combination of vocational skills, add a costume of candy-striped dolphin shorts and Swarovski-crystal-dotted tank tops, and voilà! A nation was inspired to run like hell. And count calories as they ran.

Labels that we take for granted today were not institutionalized until the Nutrition Labeling and Education Act of 1990, the year I turned ten. What had been voluntary became mandatory: disclosure of nutritional values, including saturated and unsaturated fat, sugar, and sodium, on all manufactured foods and the top-twenty selling fruits, vegetables, fish, and shellfish at any given grocery store. Meat, poultry, and egg products were addressed in 1993 with legislation coauthored by the Department of Agriculture.

Because much of the consumer activism was driven by concerns over scams related to the burgeoning diet-food market, the act focused on standardizing definitions for terms such as *low*, *lean*, *lite*, and *reduced*. Some notable exemptions to the labeling requirements were made for foods that weren't seen as contributing to the rapidly expanding waistlines of the masses. These included some infant formulas, mom-and-pop products with less than $500,000 in retail sales each year, and "spices, flavorings, and colors."

This last exception did not raise much objection at the time. Making collective declarations of something like "Cajun spice" seemed like a pragmatic nod toward minor ingredients. A set of measuring spoons doesn't include the measurements for a pinch, a dash, or a smidge. Similarly, an exception was made for incidental additives and processing aids. These loopholes would soon become troublesome.

By 1996, the FDA issued an "Allergy Warning Letter" after receiving a number of reports "concerning consumers who experienced adverse reactions following exposure to allergenic substances in foods." The culprits? Just to name a few: "natural flavorings" wherein the flavors included butter; a "processing aid" of margarine used to grease a baking sheet; tiny flakes of egg or shrimp in Japanese spice mixes.

The letter, authored by Fred Shank, director of the Center

for Food Safety and Applied Nutrition, declared that manufacturers had "incorrectly interpreted what constitutes an insignificant level of a substance." Although it was true that unlisted incidental additives could include subingredients, any additives serving a functional purpose in the final product should be listed. So if the breading on a frozen fish filet uses egg as a binder, it is not sufficient to list "bread crumbs" on the ingredients; "egg whites" needs to appear as well. Shank urged manufacturers to declare within its ingredient list any color, flavor, or spice known to be a common allergen.

In the case of Communion wafers, ritualized ingestion places religious leaders and those with allergies on opposite sides of the food fight. But in the fight for accurate food labeling, those with allergies have recognized allies among those religions that require avoidance of foods such as pork (for kosher Jews or Muslims) and beef (for Hindus). Long before ingredient lists were brought up to today's standard of specificity, my mother would remind me to look for the pareve symbol as shorthand for "dairy-free," and to beware packaged boxes marked *D*.

In a widely circulated 2003 *Daf Hakashrus* article by Rabbi Gavriel Price of the Orthodox Union Ingredients Approval Registry, Rabbi Price used the example of beta-carotene to demonstrate the complexities of hidden ingredients. Beta-carotene is a yellow or orange food agent often used to color margarine. Because margarine's appearance is not reflected in a final product, such as cookies, beta-carotene was regarded as an incidental additive and did not have to be listed under existing guidelines. But the water-dispersible variation of beta-carotene uses gelatin that could be made from fish, pork, or beef. The possibility of contamination by pork or nonkosher slaughtered beef renders the food impermissible for those who keep kosher.

(Beta-carotene is also a frequent additive to premixed juice drinks, which is why many companies invest in placing kosher pareve signs on their drink labels. For years, you'd find gelatin in Sunny Delight. They claim to have gotten rid of it when the brand relaunched as SunnyD, though they've passed on the opportunity to advertise "Now with fewer fish bones.")

Back in 2003, Rabbi Price was skeptical that the FDA would ever mandate acknowledgment of contaminating ingredients to a degree that could satisfy Jewish dietary law. In a typical processing plant, "airborne particles of whey powder, although in parts per million, can nevertheless be present in food. . . . Labeling laws do not require such declaration because the whey powder is present at 'insignificant levels.'" He judged that "the dairy or non-kosher status of equipment, important in an evaluation of the kosher or pareve status of a food, is totally outside the FDA's universe of concern."

"Totally outside the universe" proved to be a slight overstatement. In 2003, skyrocketing levels of celiac disease and peanut allergy were already shifting the mainstream perception of what constituted "insignificant levels" of exposure. Just over a year after the article in *Daf Hakashrus*, the U.S. government passed the Food Allergen Labeling and Consumer Protection Act of 2004. This act required that the secretary of Health and Human Services submit a congressional report analyzing "the ways in which foods, during manufacturing and processing, are unintentionally contaminated with major food allergens." The secretary was also instructed to begin conducting inspections to ensure the reduction or elimination of cross contact between foods. It might not have been a banishing of whey from the factory, Rabbi Price, but it was a start.

The act's primary function is to formally recognize those eight major foods or food groups that account for more than 90 percent of food allergies in the United States: milk, egg, peanuts, tree nuts, fish, shellfish, soy, and wheat. When it comes to the "big eight," loopholes have been sewn tight. Their presence may not be generalized within colorings, spices, or flavors. If a derivative such as casein is used, the label must include the major allergen label, either in the form of *casein (MILK)* or by appending *CONTAINS MILK* to the end of the ingredient list. The specific member of an allergen group must be specified; e.g., "cashews," rather than simply "nuts." Soy lecithin, used to coat baking pans, is no longer a hidden "processing aid." Provisions are made for research into national prevalence rates of food allergies and anaphylactic reactions, and to develop allergen-free guidelines for food preparation in restaurants, grocery store delicatessens, and school cafeterias.

The wheels of bureaucracy—even after they begin turning—take a long time to move the cart forward. FALCPA, as the food-allergen labeling act is sometimes called, prescribes a somewhat labyrinthine system of ingredient parsing. A year earlier, Congress had also passed a stringent set of guidelines for labeling trans fats. Out of consideration for companies absorbing the cost of rejiggering recipes and reprinting labels on dozens of products, accommodating both sets of guidelines, the FDA did not demand compliance on either front until January 1, 2006.

In February 2006, the media picked up on the fact that the

McDonald's corporation had added the phrase "contains wheat and milk ingredients" to the nutritional labeling of their French fries. The Associated Press contacted Cathy Kapica, McDonald's then director of global nutrition (a rather idealistic job title coming from the folks behind McNuggets). Kapica confirmed that a flavoring agent in the cooking oil contained "wheat and dairy derivatives." She was quick to clarify that the derivatives did not include proteins, and suggested that people with wheat or dairy allergies who had eaten fries without problem should continue eating them.

"Technically there are no allergens in there," she said. "What this is is an example of science evolving."

Uh-huh. This was not the first controversy over McDonald's flagship product. In 1990, the company had announced a switch from cooking with beef tallow to pure vegetable oil. But a 2002 lawsuit brought on by vegetarian groups revealed most fries were still being cooked in "beef-flavored oil" (to the horror of Hindus everywhere), resulting in a $10 million settlement. Apparently, McDonald's subsequent promise to *really* change the recipe had become mired in production purgatory. The reality was that they were scared to alter the taste of an iconic product; as Colonel Sanders could have attested, there would be no going back.

Watching these news reports in 2006, I didn't know whether to laugh or to cry. I didn't have many food rituals as a child. What I had were usually weird variations on what the "normal kids" did, merely offering the comfort of routine rather than signaling membership in their ranks. Who else lined up twelve hazelnuts in the pencil groove of her desk? Who else equated catching a cold with eating whole artichokes in home-brewed broth, instead of the comforting, canned conformity of Campbell's chicken noodle soup?

But I had one ritual that had made me feel like every other kid. During the first decade of my life, when I was undergoing weekly shots, only one reward brought any consolation: a trip to the McDonald's near my allergist's office. It was a particularly fancy one, with an indoor merry-go-round populated by Grimace, the Hamburglar, Birdie the Early Bird, and Ronald himself. I always knew what I would order: French fries in a cheery red cup.

Every week, I endured injections to protect me from my dairy allergy. And apparently, every week my reward had been tainted with beef.

Maybe the exposure was minimal. Just as KFC managers altered the "secret recipe" on-site, perhaps the manager of that McDonald's used vegetable oil earlier than most. Still, we should have suspected something. There were times when the fries upset my stomach, my body refusing to digest the grease and stranding me in the bathroom for twenty minutes at a time. We'd blame it on contamination by a neighboring hamburger. We all ignored the warnings, even my watchful parents.

What can I say? It was my ritual, and ritual is a powerful thing.

CHAPTER FOUR

The Great Peanut Scare

Betrayed by McDonald's, I had spent my teens and twenties searching for the next great fast-food fry. Wendy's fries are too bland. Arby's fries, though temptingly curly, are cooked in enough soybean oil to make my stomach churn. Then, thanks to my then boyfriend's weekly pilgrimages for his bacon cheese-burger, I discovered Five Guys: hand-cut, skin-on potatoes doled out with an extra scoop that guarantees copious soggy, salty, bottom-of-the-bag fry perfection.

On my first visit, I'd noticed a plaque on the front door warning guests that peanuts are served in bulk at every Five Guys—a barrel of nuts in their shells that sits by the register, available to customers to snack on while waiting for their order. I didn't think twice about it. But on my next visit, someone had taped an ink-jet, large-font sign proclaiming DUE TO THE

POSSIBILITY OF SEVERE ALLERGIC REACTION IN SOME NEIGHBOR-
HOOD CHILDREN, PLEASE DO NOT TAKE PEANUTS OR PEANUT
SHELLS OUTSIDE OF FIVE GUYS. That got my attention.

More and more, public venues show an awareness of peanut
allergies. The Washington Nationals (along with the Red Sox,
Padres, Mariners, and several other major-league teams) designate peanut-free seating zones at a couple of baseball games
each season. Sometimes a whole stadium goes peanut free for
a minor-league game—no roasted nuts, no peanut M&M's, no
Snickers. Bags are inspected at the door for contraband.

Peanut bans are spreading like cultural kudzu. No more
making peanut butter–pinecone bird feeders in kindergarten.
No more baskets of peanuts at the bar. In 2009, the Wisconsin
Division of State Facilities sent a letter to downtown offices in
Madison requesting that locals no longer feed peanuts to the
squirrels. The front lawn of the capitol had become littered with
shells, and officials feared reactions among the thousands of
children coming through for tours.

Why all the worry? Allergies among children are on the rise,
and allergies to peanuts in particular. In a study titled "Food
Allergy Among Children in the United States," published in the
November 2009 *Pediatrics*, a survey of 2005–2006 medical
records revealed a 9 percent incidence rate for peanut-sensitive
IgE antibodies. Note: This doesn't mean 9 percent of children
are allergic to peanuts. Only an oral food challenge reveals if
the antibodies actually react. But it's a marked increase from
previous levels of sensitivity.

Some try to dismiss these figures as an inflated product of
the yuppie imagination. Come Halloween, the kid who dies
"from a hidden peanut" has replaced the kid who dies "from

a razor blade hidden in the apple" in the pantheon of suburban myth. Yet in urban areas, the incidence rate of allergies is also rising. In that same 2009 study, blood samples among African-American children showed they were twice as likely as white children to carry an IgE antibody for peanuts. The Hispanic population, though exhibiting the lowest prevalence rate overall, showed the greatest increase from previous years.

In an interview for *Living Without* (a magazine that caters to those with food allergies, celiac disease, and other dietary restrictions), Jackie Clegg Dodd—wife of U.S. senator Christopher Dodd and mother of two children, including Grace, a child with multiple food sensitivities—recounted an experience that epitomizes the extreme scenarios associated with peanut allergies:

> One time I was flying with Gracie and her baby sister and the airline rep informed passengers that they couldn't eat tree nuts and peanuts during the flight. As we were taking off, the woman seated behind me threw a fit about it. I offered to share lunch with her grandchild—I'd packed plenty of great food—but she declined. Then as we were beginning descent, she gave her grandchild a peanut butter and jelly sandwich. Within minutes, Gracie was projectile vomiting. There I was alone, nursing one baby while the other was going into severe anaphylaxis. When the plane landed, we went straight to the hospital.

Clearly, the PB&J-smuggling granny is the bad guy in this story. Yet I find myself nagging at what is known, and what is implied. What does Dodd think was the reaction catalyst? Was it the smell of the peanut butter? Peanut oil contact-transferred up to their row in a matter of minutes? Isn't it more likely that the child ingested an old crumb in the area of her seat, or that one of her own snacks was contaminated?

What if that woman's grandchild had allergies of her own? I think of all the times a peanut butter sandwich or peanut butter pretzels served as my anchor for a long trip. Even a supposedly allergy-friendly in-flight meal usually arrives with a fat slice of cucumber in the salad and cost-friendly cantaloupe mixed among the fruit. There's something slightly self-righteous in Dodd's offer of her "great food." I imagine someone offering my mother a package of Garden Salsa (and whey-laced) Sun Chips instead, or a home-baked brownie, with the presumption that it will be a welcome option for her hungry child. The exchange would not go well.

I've heard advocates for nut-free zones say "anyone can live without nuts for [a meal, a ball game, a flight]." That's true, I guess. But what if every one of the "big eight" allergen contingents demanded the same courtesy, every time? Do those who want public spheres to be free of egg or dairy or shellfish have any less right to the safety of their children than those who want protection from nuts?

The same 2009 study that demonstrated a 9 percent prevalence rate of peanut-sensitive antibodies revealed a 12 percent prevalence rate of antibodies respondent to milk. There are multiple times I've had reactions in a movie theater upon sitting too close to someone with buttered popcorn. My eyes blur, and I begin to wheeze. But it would have never occurred to my folks to lobby theater owners to designate popcorn-free shows. On an airplane, it is true that I blanch when someone sits down with a bag from California Pizza Kitchen. For the next few hours, I'll lean in the opposite direction to breathe, and make sure my seatmate's oily napkins don't land on my lap tray. But I can't imagine requiring a pizza-free flight.

Why is a generation of children being raised under the belief that it takes a village to avoid a peanut?

. . .

"Kids don't want to feel different," asserts Jenny Kales, a Chicago writer, mother of two, and author of *The Nut-Free Mom* blog. We're on the phone, talking about the challenges of raising a child with food allergies. She is determined to make her daughter feel protected without setting her apart. Neither Kales nor her husband has allergies of their own. So when their child Alexandra first seemed to be repelled by nut-based foods, beginning in early childhood, "we thought it was just her preference."

Then, in 2004, a teacher forced the four-year-old to try a bite of the peanut butter and jelly sandwiches being served in her preschool facility. At the end of the school session, Kales arrived to find her daughter had swollen eyes and hives. She asked why she had not been called and was told, "You were about to pick her up anyway." The school officials suggested Alexandra might have an undiagnosed allergy. While Kales was driving to the store to buy Benadryl, her daughter began exhibiting anaphylaxis. Alexandra vomited and fainted.

"I've never in my life seen anything like that," Kales remembers. Though Alexandra had seemed "perfectly healthy" up to that point, testing confirmed IgE sensitivity to peanuts and tree nuts. The family began changing their lifestyle to keep her safe—starting with transferring her to a preschool more careful about allergies.

Many educators don't think about the thousand little ways food substances can sneak into the school day. Wheat makes an appearance in Play-Doh; egg is often used in tempera paints. Someone's well-meaning donation of moisturizing soap might feature soy proteins, cucumber additives, or cashew oil.

Take Elmer's glue. It may be dairy free now, but for years it used casein (a milk derivative) as a binder. Small wonder, given that the parent company, Borden, was primarily in the dairy-product business. Elsie the Cow was a real cow, purchased in Connecticut and subsequently promoted as Borden's unofficial mascot. Her "husband" was a bull named Elmer, who became the mascot of Borden's chemical division. Hence, Elmer's glue.

Kales has become what she calls a "food detective," always on the lookout for hidden dangers. She uses her blog to share her findings with the larger community of allergy moms, posting two to three times a week on media coverage of medical research, tips for surviving the holidays, and reviews of the latest nut-free product brands. Unfortunately, manufacturing trends for the food-allergic sometimes pit those with different sensitivities against one another. As more parents are trying to protect their children from wheat allergies or celiac disease, gluten-free baking products—which often use nut flour as a substitute— are popping up everywhere.

"I am terrified by gluten-free," Kales says. Nut flour is a growing problem in restaurants as well. When it comes to family outings, they rarely grab a meal unannounced. Kales calls first to speak with a manager and make sure her daughter can be accommodated.

"You lose a lot of life's spontaneity," she admits.

Kales finds it easier to keep a nut-free household, rather than risk accidental contamination. My mother did not keep milk in our fridge for the same reason; for years, my parents gave up blue-cheese dressing on salads.

For his workday lunches, Kales's husband sometimes "cheats" by indulging in peanut-laden Thai food. That means being quarantined from contact with his daughter until he's had a chance to fully wash up.

"Alexandra asks him, 'Why would you get that?,'" Kales says. I understand her daughter's sense of betrayal, especially at the age of ten. I felt the same way when my father used to buy strawberry milkshakes at the drive-through.

In order to continue keeping their daughter away from nuts, the family found an elementary school that allows the children to go home for lunch. But there is a trade-off for this freedom; when Alexandra wants to stay, there is no peanut-free table, as there are at some schools. No matter how carefully she seats herself, the migratory habits of kids in a lunchroom make it impossible to prevent exposure.

Remembering the many times I ended up in the school clinic, and thinking of all the horror stories one hears about peanut sensitivity, I ask how bad her reactions have gotten. Her mother's answer shocks me, but not in the way I expect. In the five years since Alexandra's diagnosis, and given what Kales acknowledged have been "extreme lifestyle changes," the number of subsequent anaphylactic reactions has been: zero. None.

I've got the phone cocked to my ear as Kales is talking about how her daughter's face broke out in a rash after eating some Chinese noodles—in other words, evidence that her tree-nut allergy is still a real threat, even if it's never been witnessed in a confirmed anaphylactic moment. I'm listening. But mainly I'm transfixed by the realization that this family thinks in terms of *the* reaction. One episode that set off a complete lifestyle change. One episode that might define a year.

I grew up thinking in terms of not *the* reaction, but *a* reaction, perhaps as many as one a week. Trial and error has been my way of life. It's not that my parents were negligent; they just had a different understanding of what my options were.

"Why have a problem with a peanut-free table?" Kales asks. Though she does not support school peanut bans—"it's not practical"—she wishes cafeterias would refrain from actively selling nut-based foods. And she's relieved that their school has prohibited birthday treats across the board. "No one gets them; it's not just my daughter."

I ask what she thinks about airplanes. Kales pauses, and in that pause I hear the hesitation of many allergy moms: *Do I speak in terms of my child and my experience? Or am I hoisting a banner for all allergic children?*

She references the work of Dr. Hugh Sampson, director of the Jaffe Food Allergy Institute, to explain the danger of the mile-high environment. Allergic reactions are triggered by exposure to proteins. During the pulverizing and sorting processes common to the manufacture of many single-serving foods, proteins become powdered and cling to the inside of the package. If you've ever licked your finger and swept it along the inside crease of a potato chip bag, you know what I'm talking about. The air in a plane's cabin is both pressurized and recirculated, so that nut residue has nowhere to go once released. As Dr. Sampson's work has suggested, the residue can reach critical mass when dozens of passengers open packages all at once.

A frequently cited 1996 Mayo Clinic study showed significant accumulations of nut protein in the air filters of many commercial planes. This study, like many in the allergy world, suffered from a relatively small sample size—two planes, each of which had logged five thousand hours of flight since its last filter change. But the meager evidence, combined with the pressure of advocacy groups, has been enough to convince the Department of Transportation to investigate the possibility of establishing peanut-free zones on passenger airlines or banning airline distribution of peanuts entirely.

Some companies have acquiesced, including American Airlines and Northwest Airlines, which switched to pretzels. Others are holdouts; Southwest Airlines considers nuts, served in a package proclaiming "Byte-sized Fares," an important part of its market positioning. Since their low-overhead structure also includes open seating, Southwest officials have argued that buffer zones would be impossible to secure. Sometimes the decision is made by the politics of the business. When Delta—not coincidentally headquartered in Atlanta, Georgia, a peanut production capital—acquired Northwest Airlines in 2009, peanuts returned to NWA flights.

I get that people with allergies would rather avoid the risk of itchy eyes, a runny nose, and the emotional drain. What I don't get are the people pitching it as a scenario of life or death. Airborne reactions are real. Anaphylaxis is real. But it's as if the mainstream media, becoming aware of the two around the same time, melded them as one phenomenon: airborne anaphylaxis. And a generation of parents have convinced themselves this hybrid is a legitimate and pervasive threat. Really?

"Our doctor has mentioned it is a misnomer," Kales says when I ask for her take. "We don't worry about it too much."

Even as a nut-free mom, she is skeptical of parents who claim their children have had severe reactions to the smell of an allergen. She should be. Scent is carried by pyrazines, organic compounds that stimulate the mucous membranes of your nose (and are also responsible for shaping flavor). These chemicals are fundamentally different from proteins. So until the model of allergic reactions changes, there is no way a smell alone can trigger an IgE-based reaction.

What a smell *could* trigger is a psychosomatic reaction based on the conditioning of past experience. Symptoms such as rashes, hives, vomiting, and rapid fluctuations in blood pressure, temperature, or respiration—all these symptoms are indicative of allergic reactions, and all are phenomena that laboratory subjects have been shown capable of manifesting in response to nothing more than sufficiently stressful situations. I'm not saying that these reactions should be dismissed; they have to be treated immediately, on the presumption that they are IgE based. But when backtracking later to identify the origin of a reaction, it is important to open your mind to all the possibilities.

Once, my parents took me to Hersheypark in Pennsylvania. I'd begged to go, but upon arriving found the constant references to milk and milk chocolate a little creepy. I didn't want to be greeted by people dressed as foil-covered Kisses. I couldn't have any of the free samples. Boarding one roller coaster, I overheard someone say that we would swing over Chocolate World, the on-site candy factory.

I became certain, *certain*, that a puff of milk-laced exhaust would kill me. But it was too late. I was strapped in. As we rounded a sharp curve, we entered a pocket of air that seemed particularly heavy with the stink of chocolate. My small, adrenaline-filled body tensed up. My face felt hot. I began to wheeze. I got off the ride in tears, went straight for my inhaler, and spent the rest of the afternoon in the refuge of the carousel.

For years I described this incident as another one of my allergy attacks. I suppose there's a thousand minor ways I could have been exposed to milk proteins during the day. But I don't think that was the culprit. Not this time. I was a fearful child, self-consciously primed to have a reaction, and so I did.

Honest discussion of these types of reactions—which might help us bridge the gap between what is viscerally experienced and what is medically justifiable—is stifled in the allergic community. We feel like we can't afford to give up any ground, because some want to believe almost *all* allergic reactions are psychosomatic.

In an infamous January 2009 *Los Angeles Times* op-ed column, Joel Stein called allergies a "yuppie invention." He was drawing on an essay in the *British Medical Journal,* by Harvard University sociologist Dr. Nicholas Christakis, on the notion of contagious anxiety. It didn't help when *Time* magazine, in an article published that same month, quoted Christakis as using the term *mass panic* to describe the attitudes of many parents and school officials toward food allergies.

The reaction was, well, mass outrage. Dr. Robert A. Wood,

a professor of pediatrics at Johns Hopkins University School of Medicine, published a *Los Angeles Times* rejoinder calling Stein's column "insulting and inappropriate."

Yet he did not entirely disagree with Christakis. The impetus for Christakis's original *BMJ* commentary was an incident of a bus being evacuated in the Massachusetts school district where one of his own children attended classes. Why the evacuation? A peanut found on the bus floor. These weren't preschoolers unable to discern a threat or keep their hands out of their mouths. These were ten-year-olds. Wood acknowledged that for that age, zero tolerance is probably an unnecessary precaution.

"It's an unfortunate situation," Wood told Tiffany Sharples, the *Time* reporter, "if a family with an inaccurate perception of the allergy leads a child to believe that a Snickers bar from fifty feet away is a lethal weapon."

There must be a compromise between the cavalier and puritanical. Right?

"There's something about peanuts and peanut butter that makes people crazy—on both sides," Jenny Kales warned me. "Peanut butter is iconic, so strongly associated with childhood. Banning it is seen as anti-American."

For the peanut farmers, this isn't just a matter of patriotism; their livelihoods are at stake. Every store or institution that bans peanuts hurts business. So does every peanut-related death that circulates in the news.

In March 2000, Dee Dee Darden founded the National Peanut Board (NPB), a representative body for peanut farmers. The board's activities, which focus on scientific research, domestic advertising, and export promotion, are funded through a 1 percent assessment levied on annual peanut crop values. Soon after the board's formation, Darden approached the council's leaders with a radical idea: to fund not just agricultural science but research into the explosive rise of peanut allergies.

"We faced a lot of opposition at first, especially from those in the industry," Darden says. "They thought if we talked about it too much, it made it a forefront issue."

Darden was determined. "I'd heard all the numbers," she tells me. "We wanted to have a positive impact on the situation." Darden, then in her early forties, had grown up in a farming family of Suffolk—"there wasn't hardly a day I wasn't out in the dirt"—in a region of Virginia once referred to as the peanut capital of the world. "It was hard to believe. I never knew anyone who had any allergies, much less peanut allergies . . . but we didn't want to be ostriches, with our heads in the sand."

Darden and her colleagues wondered where their relatively small amount of start-up money could make the most difference. So they created the Scientific Advisory Council (SAC), a rotating panel of five leading doctors and scientists from the United States, Canada, and the United Kingdom. Though each member is already prominent in the field of allergy study, the SAC's biannual meetings bring them together for brainstorming sessions, for the opportunity to share research results, and to decide which proposals the NPB should offer future grant support.

"They were like little children, all excited to be in the same room," Darden remembers. "You know, like when children's faces light up? We were a bunch of peanut farmers, putting all these great minds together."

In the past ten years, the SAC has overseen the cumulative allocation of nearly $7 million of NPB funding for allergy study and education. One vein of research looks at which peanut-preparation techniques release the most proteins. On a molecular level, it turns out that dry roasted peanuts are more "allergic" than ones that have been boiled. This may explain why frequency of peanut reaction is so high in the United States, where dry roasting is the norm, even in the production of peanut butter. In China, where peanut consumption is comparable but the peanuts are steamed or boiled, the incidence of allergy is low.

Scientific data is a double-edged sword. Some discoveries are welcome to peanut farmers; others make their jobs harder. One focal point for investigation has been defining the minimum exposure capable of eliciting a reaction. The latest research suggests the threshold is about one-tenth of one peanut, a frighteningly small amount for farmers when negotiating with manufacturers wary of cross-contamination at processing plants. Scientists have also shown that peanut oil can be refined to the point that the reactive proteins are removed, resulting in FDA approval to take that refined oil off the "allergen" list (this is also true of some soy oils)—great news for farmers. But complicating matters is the reality that this process has a higher price point than cold-pressed, expeller-pressed, or extruded peanut oil.

One study funded in part by the SAC looked at the degree to which peanut proteins are passed from mother to child via breast milk. For many years, parents have been advised to avoid exposing their children to peanuts until the age of two. Did breast-feeding mothers need to abstain from peanuts as well? Then, in October 2009, *Pediatrics* published a study demonstrating a correlation between early consumption of peanuts and a *low* incidence of peanut allergy. The American Academy of Pediatrics has changed their official stance and recommends that peanuts be administered to children whenever parents judge developmentally appropriate.

Peanut farmers aren't rejoicing just yet. It's one thing to get a vote of confidence at the organizational level. It's another thing to get thousands of local doctors, used to telling new mothers one thing, to start telling them another.

I call up Ryan Lepicier, the NPB director of communications, who works to reconcile the advice of the scientific community with ingrained local policies. He reaches out to schools struggling to formulate their peanut- and other allergen-related protocols. Each time, he says, he must first figure out who is driving the decisions. The principal? The dietician? The school board? The parents? Lepicier sees the decision to ban some foods outright—a policy, he is quick to note, not endorsed by such groups as the Food Allergy and Anaphylaxis Network— as part of a slippery slope in which lobbying and political correctness trump common sense.

"It's like the association of nurses," he recalls, "who didn't want to implement programs fighting obesity because students would be 'singled out.' Or schools that didn't serve grapes because the janitors didn't want to clean them up off the floor."

The National Peanut Board has an undeniable financial stake in avoiding peanut bans. But Lepicier hopes that as Americans learn more from international allergy studies, the NPB will no longer have to be its own best advocate. In 2008, a team headed by Dr. Gideon Lack announced that in a study looking at ten thousand Jewish children (i.e., a cohort with genetic similarity), those who had been raised in London were about ten times more likely to have peanut sensitivity than those raised in Tel Aviv. Lack theorized that one contributing factor could be the predominance of Israeli children exposed to peanuts via a popular peanut-based treat, Bamba.

First debuted in the mid-1960s, Bamba is corn that is puffed, enriched with vitamins, and sprayed with Argentinean peanut butter before it cools. Picture a peanut-based equivalent of a Cheez Doodle. An even sweeter "strawberry" version is also available, dyed red with beetroot. It's a ubiquitous treat in Israel, often fed to toddlers as their first finger food.

Lack theorized that tykes chewing on Bamba were somehow inoculating themselves against peanut allergy. In contrast, the widespread Western timeline of "protecting" children under age three from peanut exposure might be contributing to peanut allergy, instead of preventing it. With grant support from several groups including the NPB and the National Institutes of Health, Lack has launched the LEAP (Learning Early About Peanut Allergy) Study, an ambitious seven-year study that has enrolled 640 children, all between the ages of four months and ten months, considered at high risk for peanut allergy because of diagnosed eczema or egg allergy. Half of these children will be restricted from peanut exposure; half will be exposed regularly between the ages of ten months and three years. When the participants reach the age of five, they will be tested for peanut allergy.

This data, which should become available in 2014, will primarily impact attitudes toward prenatal and early childhood peanut exposure. But it may also persuasively align with shifting attitudes toward treating established peanut allergies through low-level exposure rather than absolute avoidance. That is, pending the success of oral immunotherapy approaches only now being attempted. These breakthroughs glimmer as part of a more rational future.

In the meantime, we have entrepreneurs like Sharon Perry, co-owner of the Southern Star Ranch Boarding Kennel in Florence, Texas. Perry has devoted a division of her corporation to the cultivation of service animals taught to detect peanuts. Their proponents hope these companions will become as widely accepted as seeing-eye dogs. Perry claims to screen three hundred candidates for every single dog chosen for the program. Once you factor in purchase, vaccinations, and up to six months of training, the price of one of these dogs can top ten thousand dollars. In one promotional video, I watched a harnessed Labrador walk up the aisle of a public library with his master, stopping at any book that had once been handled by a child's nut-contaminated fingertips.

I ask Lepicier what the European scientists he works with think of America's peanut-sniffing dogs.

"They are aghast," he says.

. . .

When allergies come up in conversation, I hear one of two comments. The first is "Oh, I know a person who is so allergic to [fill in the blank]." The second is "The schools now—you can't serve anything. It's unbelievable!" Those uttering the latter follow with a guilty look, as if I won't understand. But I do. In an effort to protect children, we've asked everyone to join us in the briar patch. Parenting is hard enough without having to reinvent the sandwich, just for the sake of your kid's classmate.

So people call the situation "unbelievable." As in, "I can't believe the change from when I was a child." Or as in, "I can't believe this is all really necessary."

In the gap between what is feared and what is believed, folks have accumulated hostility toward those of us who claim severe allergies. You find skepticism in the comment boards for allergy-centric op-ed pieces, where anonymous voices suggest it's all in our heads, that we're making others abet our neuroses. You can hear the resentment in pockets of the restaurant industry. One Las Vegas chef told Ryan Lepicier, "Some people say they have an allergy when they just don't want to eat something."

Something is awry when the news delivers stories like the 2007 incident in which a janitor at the Riverside Bakery in Nottingham, England, purposefully strewed peanuts around the facility—usually a nut-free zone—after being disciplined for putting a calendar of nude girls up on the wall. The bakery, part of a larger plant called Pork Farms, estimated that they lost $1.6 million in delayed production while decontaminating the factory. *Janitor Goes Nuts*, says the link to the story I find online.

If the story was arsenic being thrown around a baby food jarring facility, no one would be laughing. Yet we do laugh. More and more, food allergies are being played in movies and television for laughs.

I grew up watching *The Simpsons*, and there's a season-eighteen episode in which Bart (newly revealed to have a shrimp allergy) and Principal Skinner (newly revealed to have a peanut allergy) face off on the landing of a Thai food factory in the previously unknown Little Bangkok section of Springfield. Their weapons? A peanut tied to the end of one long stick, a shrimp tied to the end of another. The sound track? "Duel of the Fates" from *Star Wars* lightsaber battles. Their fight comes to a draw when the catwalk collapses, dumping them into a vat of equally imperiling peanut-covered shrimp. And I laughed, I did. I can take a joke.

But *The Simpsons* is, by definition, a cartoonish treatment of the world. What worries me are the programs that do not operate in the register of satire or surrealism. These shows develop a grounded setting, present three-dimensional characters, and invest in those characters' emotions; yet when the plotline employs an allergy incident, it does so with callousness that suggests the writers don't see allergies as any real threat to life.

The media frames food allergies with three recurring clichés. The first cliché: the allergic reaction as sight gag. In *Hitch*, a 2005 romantic comedy, Will Smith plays matchmaker Alex "Hitch" Hitchens, and Eva Mendes costars as his love interest. When Hitch accidentally ingests shellfish, his eyelids swell into a grotesque mask. This isn't a way of showing that Hitch's braggadocio is actually rooted in a lifetime of vulnerability over whether his body can be trusted not to turn on him. Nah. This is an excuse for Smith's character to go into a drugstore, scarf down Benadryl, and stage a "look, he's acting like a funny drunk" scene, which is about as funny as the ol' runaway wheelchair gag.

The second cliché: allergy as Achilles' heel, in which an otherwise competent, competitive character is taken out by an allergen. In the ABC Family movie *Picture This*, the prototypical "evil blonde," Lisa Cross, is determined to prevent the lead character, Mandy Gilbert (played by *High School Musical* star Ashley Tisdale), from going to a party with Cross's ex-boyfriend. Her solution? She bribes a mall worker to sell Gilbert a nut-laced smoothie, knowing this will transform the allergic girl's features into the dreaded "butt face."

Three years earlier, in the big-screen *Monster-in-Law*, Jane Fonda's titular character sneaks peanuts into the Jennifer Lopez nut-allergic character's food the night before her wedding day, hoping a reaction will prevent Lopez from marrying her son. The real-world potential for a charge of attempted murder? Details, details.

The third cause for an allergy cameo: provide an excuse for the protagonist to act heroically. In the recent movie version of *Nancy Drew*, Emma Roberts's Nancy is introduced as a brave, practical, and preternaturally well-read young teen. Our proof? A party where one of Nancy's friends passes out on the floor, and it's discovered she is in the grip of an anaphylactic reaction due to a known peanut allergy.

Nobody asks if the girl carries an epinephrine injector. Instead, it just so happens that Nancy is versed in at-home tracheotomies. Give her a ballpoint pen, a pocketknife, and some room, and she can save a life. (The grateful friend appears in a later scene, remarkably none the worse for wear. There is no scarring in the world of teen cinema.)

All these clichés come together in a 2005 episode of *That's So Raven* that still lives on in syndication. I caught it one night during one of those dull-eyed, 1 a.m. moments when it's either the Disney Channel or HGTV, and I'd already seen that episode of *Property Virgins*. So instead I got season three's "Chef-Man and Raven." Victor Baxter and his daughter, Raven (played by Raven-Symoné, aka Olivia from *The Cosby Show*), are invited to compete against Victor's former college cooking rival for the *Iron Chef*–styled program *Challenge Captain Cook-off*.

When it looks as though Raven and her father have a fighting chance of defeating the defending champions, their jealous competitors take matters into their own hands by spiking Raven's dish with mushrooms. Apparently, fungi are Raven's Achilles' heel. (I suspect the only reason the scriptwriters didn't go with peanuts was that it would have been too difficult to ensure continuity; odds are that at some point in the three seasons leading up to this, her character had been shown eating a peanut butter *something*.)

Once Raven ingests the mushrooms, the camera steps into her point of view so we can see her vision is blurring. Her father notices and diagnoses an allergy attack, declaring only "this is worse than last time!" When we switch back to an outside view, we see the actress's face is layered in bubbles of fake flesh, so that her eyes are squeezed shut and her cheeks are puffed out in a parody of allergy edema. Her actual hands are encased in cartoon gloves of inflated skin. Sight gag: check.

The team knows they have been sabotaged, which makes Raven all the more determined to keep cooking. Her father, otherwise portrayed as a rational adult, okays this after a two-second hesitation. No pause for Benadryl. No mention of penalizing the opposing team. Raven's allergies are Raven's problem.

The contest comes down to Victor's ability to execute the

"quadruple flip" of a pan-fried fish. The best their competitors can accomplish is a triple. Of course, in the crucial moment (heroic action alert), his daughter must step in and complete the trick for him. She does so not in spite of her allergies but because of them. When the filet of trout looks like it might not make its last midair rotation, Raven claps her obscenely swollen cheeks and—as if expressing air from a bellows—*blows* the fish through its final turn.

When she must catch the fish to win, her pan is out of reach. No problem! She sticks out her hand, which thanks to her allergies has grown to the size of a dinner plate. She catches the sizzling fish in her bare but conveniently numbed-by-hives palm.

This is what personal victory looks like on the Disney Channel.

This isn't late-night sketch comedy. This is not an art house film. The bottom line is a big issue for shows like this one. If anyone thought there would be enough outcry to injure an actor's brand or lead to a boycott, scenes would have been rewritten. They were not. Actors, directors, screenwriters, producers, and dozens of others sign off on these projects before they make it to the screen.

The good news about all the activity galvanized by those with peanut allergies is that we've become a blip on the cultural radar. The bad news is that food allergies have the dubious honor of having joined a long line of diseases—gout, asthma, chronic fatigue syndrome—for which that blip doubles as a moving target.

CHAPTER FIVE

King Soy and the Body Politic

So much rides on empathy, at the end of the day. Mothers find (or fail to find) a way to relate to their allergic children. A classmate forgoes his peanut butter sandwich so he can sit with his best friend at the nut-free table in the school cafeteria. You'd think, given all the times I rely on empathy from the world around me—from teacher to chef to airline stewardess—I'd have a heightened empathetic instinct of my own.

You'd be wrong. When my eleven-year-old sister announced that she had decided to become a vegetarian, I didn't applaud her philosophical stance. I didn't look forward to commiserating over restaurants that couldn't (or wouldn't) accommodate her. Instead, I thought, *Of course. Of course, when I would give anything to have her options, she voluntarily gives them away.*

The little snot.

From the vantage point of being ten years older, I thought Christina's choice of a meatless diet was a self-indulgence, no more rational than the six months when, at age three, her favorite snack was Heinz ketchup dipped out of a bowl with her bare finger.

Her vegetarian stance would later complicate a trip to Fort Worth, Texas, for the Beasley "cousins" reunion. My father was going back as something of a hometown hero, to share pictures and stories of his troops. The army had promoted him through various leadership roles all the way up to brigadier general, commanding army reserve soldiers in six of the largest Midwestern states. My childhood had been peppered by periods when he had returned to active duty, then deployed.

It had been years since our family had visited Texas, back before Christina had even been born. I recalled the seven-year-old me's impression of Houston: a hangar-sized warehouse with BINGO painted on its silver roof (which surely housed row after row of gaming grandmas, as far as the eye could see); the smell of cigarette smoke laced with spicy Shalimar perfume; winning an oversized pink bear at the Six Flags amusement park; chatting with surprised truckers via Grandpa Joe's CB radio.

The flight from Washington, D.C., to Dallas's Love Field airport, and then the drive to Fort Worth, left us all exhausted and starving. My father parked us at the first upscale restaurant he saw on the way into town. Leaving us in the car for a few minutes, he stepped inside to speak with the manager.

He returned and assured my mother, "The chef says it's no problem."

Meaning, no problem for me. As we walked in, my mother said, "I wondered if he asked about the vegetarian options?"

We should have been tipped off by the fact that every chair in the place was upholstered in leather. Christina balked, but, realizing she didn't have a choice, we sat down. Texas: 1, Vegetarian: 0.

I had easy if limited options in the form of an appetizer of asparagus wrapped in prosciutto (west of the Mississippi, *prosciutto* means bacon), a grilled chicken breast, and a plain baked potato. Christina's options consisted of an appetizer of mixed greens, followed by a second course of more mixed greens and a plain baked potato.

She looked to me for confirmation that, yes, the salad dinner is a lousy deal. But I avoided her gaze. I was still envious of how casually she could take a corn bread muffin, along with everyone else, from the bread basket placed on the table. So I played the poor allergic girl. When my asparagus came, I adopted a joyful tone, worthy of any Dickensian orphan, at the luxury of a straight-off-the-menu appetizer.

"So good! You have to try it!" Pause. "Okay, not you, obviously."

The next day, we gathered at the house of George Marvin, a cardiologist and that year's reunion host. Beasleys are equal parts eccentric in their interests and meticulous in their craft. Our ranks include Charles, a renowned geologist and snake expert; Lola, a University of Texas at El Paso business professor emeritus whose legal blindness has not kept her from paddling the Amazon; and Ray Olachia, a full-blooded Apache who travels the state advising on flint napping and basket weaving.

We call it the "cousins" reunion because of the difficulty everyone has keeping track of how we're related. One couple that has been attending for years—she always in a floral shirt, he in a navy blue cap—has no blood tie to the family that anyone can figure out. But they're such nice people that no one can bear to question them on it.

Midmorning, as people were still arriving, George Marvin called on everyone to form a prayer circle before our first meal. Christina and I hung back until we realized that this was not an optional exercise. We joined hands, the chain of people squeezing to fit around the sofas and chairs that crowded the living room.

"Look," one of the cousins said, "we've formed a heart."

George Marvin eyed the group with a doctor's precision. "A heart with a collapsed left ventricle," he pointed out. We prayed.

When the buffet lunch was unveiled, I realized I was in serious trouble. Chips with the cheese already melted on; salad with the cucumber and egg already diced in.

"What's that?" my sister asked, though she already knew the answer, pointing to a sliver of pink nestled among the romaine.

"Ham," answered our hostess, George Marvin's longtime girlfriend.

Oh, come on, I thought, watching as my sister stiffened. My mother moved into the kitchen to scavenge for us, gathering whatever chips she could find in their original bag and whatever greens remained in the fridge.

Years before, our grandmother had gotten over her skepticism regarding my allergies. But she couldn't understand Christina's new mission, or her subsequent frustration. She looked at my sister's empty plate.

"Honey, you know God gave us animals so we could eat them," she said.

The day loped along as a series of conversations with family. We moved from hanging out in the living room to chatting on the driveway (where beer waited in someone's car trunk, hidden from Lola's disapproval), to lounging out by the pool. Ray arrived and set up his weaving under the tent that was intended for smokers. He palmed a flat disk that would serve as one basket's base, curled the rest of the reeds into a bucket of water where they could soak into pliancy, and went to work. I stayed close to him, pretending the cigarette smoke didn't make me sneeze.

My Houston memories were not serving me well. I tried to figure out which grandaunt was Ruth, and which was Elaine, but their faces blurred in recollection. Elaine, it turned out, was the woman who would later remind me with great affection, "My God, you were such an annoying little know-it-all twerp when you were seven."

With no other teens in the house, Christina took refuge in one of the several five-hundred-page paperbacks she'd crammed into her suitcase. Every invitation seemed designed to offend her vegetarian ethic. No, she didn't really want to tour the taxidermy collection. No, she'd skip the stockyard cattle drive, thanks very much.

My sister's reticence made me ever more determined to prove that I was one of the Beasleys. In the kitchen, I got into a discussion of hot salsas and bragged that I had inherited the Texan tongue. George Marvin dared me to nibble on one of the peppers growing on his windowsill. I grabbed the whole thing and popped it into my mouth. It turned out to be a Scotch bonnet, which measures about 325,000 Scoville Heat Units. A jalapeño is only 5,000 units.

My tongue felt as if I'd French-kissed an electrical socket. My eyes welled with tears. I tried to gulp water nonchalantly, which only spread the fire down my throat.

"Milk?" a cousin offered. "You know, milk's the only thing that really helps."

I shook my head and retreated, coughing, to a deck chair out back. Twenty minutes later, the pain had lessened to a dull throb. As the sun began to set, I stared blankly at the far edge of the pool and counted the number of blue-tailed skinks that ventured along its concrete lip.

After a while Christina came outside and walked back and forth along the edge, periodically dipping her toes into the water.

"So," she blurted out all of a sudden. "Dad had another wife?"

Good lord. Someone had posted an overly complete family tree by the washroom. I tried to explain that this wasn't some major branch of his past that we had hidden from her; it was barely a twig, a brief marriage with no kids. I told her how I had found out, also on my own, also at fourteen, by noticing our father was labeled *Divorced* on our parents' marriage certificate. She was not comforted.

In every family, at some point you must face your ability to disappoint one another. But our family seems to have a special knack for minor facts made major in their suppression—and the subsequent ambush of truth. Before I could find the right thing to say, we were called inside. Some of the cousins had made dinner.

"Beef brisket," the boys announced proudly, "slow cooked."

Christina and I fixed yet another plate of chips and salsa, and made a space for ourselves on the living room floor. They put on the old home movies, black-and-white reels of people I knew to be great-grandfathers and grandaunts. I wanted so badly to feel a flash of kinship. But no matter how hard I squinted, I did not recognize their faces.

The next day was better, in that funny way things improve when they can get no worse. My father took my uncle Jim, my cousin Michele, and Christina out for a day of horse riding—the one Texan tradition that didn't put animals on the receiving end of a bullet or a fork. There would be no talk of the first wife. That wasn't our way.

My mother and I stayed by the pool, until she was hijacked for a walking tour of George Marvin's clinic. Two hours later she returned with a box of rocks that Charles had sworn included agates and geodes, and her real quarry, which was a purse full of Benadryl and Allegra samples.

"Look at this!" she said. "Six months' worth."

A pool volleyball game started up, complete with the ninety-four-year-old Lola in her polka-dot swimsuit. The horse riders returned. Dinner plans were announced: leftover brisket and cold-cut sandwiches.

Day three of survival eating. If I had one more corn chip, I was going to throw up. My mother disassembled a sandwich, peeling the turkey away to make a cheese sandwich for Christina. She pieced together one last, limp salad for me out of the lettuce and tomatoes that had been set aside for the sandwiches.

Watching Mom bustle from counter to counter, I realized

that Christina and I weren't the only ones struggling. She was, after all, a Pruett in a house full of Beasleys. There was quiet ferocity in the way she ripped iceberg into fork-friendly chunks. Fending for her daughters gave her a mission.

Before the annual white-elephant gift exchange that closed each reunion, my father showed slides from his army work: action shots in Afghanistan, mudslides he had surveyed in Honduras, flag ceremonies at Fort Snelling, and Norman, the nineteen-hand horse gifted to the Blue Devils Horse Platoon by the queen of England. The family clapped with a sincerity that's hard to come by in D.C., where people are quick to think of patriotism as a political strategy rather than a priority. In Texas, when people thank you for "serving our country," they mean it. Ray presented handwoven baskets to my mother, then me, then Christina, thanking us for our service as well.

The mood of the gift exchange was giddy; what one Beasley wanted, another stole. No one really seemed to mind. The gifts ranged from exotic textiles to doilies to pens to pocketknives. I finagled my way into possession of a small toy station wagon, in the style I recognized from the home movies of the night before.

Christina ended up with a plaster frog, pale green, easily eight inches tall and flashing a beatific grin. Was it intended as a paperweight? A lawn ornament? It was hideous, but hideous in all the right ways. She smiled and patted the head of her new pet.

Watching her, I realized that her need to be The Vegetarian, even in a roomful of barbecue lovers, was selfish only in a world that revolves around food allergies. My world has to have that focus on food allergies. Hers should not. I tapped her on the knee.

"What are you going to name the frog?" I asked.

A plane ride later, the first morning back was amiably jet-lagged. While my sister slept in, my mother cooked bacon for the omnivores. We got to work unzipping suitcases.

"Oh!" my mother called out from our kitchen. "Oh no."

Despite careful packing amid Tupperware and towels, Christina's frog had lost its feet in the jostling of baggage claim. My parents and I surveyed the wreckage of dust and once-webbed plaster. How could we break it to her? After four days and a cross-country trip, the family finally shared a common interest, in one immediate and unspoken decision.

"I did see those on sale at Rite Aid last week," my mother said.

"I'll get the car," said my dad.

. . .

From tattoos to ritual fasts, humans have long used the canvas of their bodies to display tribal, religious, cultural, and political affiliations. The practice of vegetarianism can be traced to ancient eras. The Jains in the sixth century BCE preached nonviolence toward animals. Ashoka the Great, a Buddhist emperor who ruled in second-century BCE India, formally outlawed sacrifice and hunting and ensured that even "cocks are not to be caponized, and husks hiding living beings are not to be burnt."

In classical antiquity, the Greek term for vegetarianism

translated to "abstinence from beings with a soul." In southern Italy, avoiding meat was admired as following the "Pythagorean way of life." (Not to be confused with believing that the square of your hypotenuse equals the sum of the squares of your other two sides.)

Monks of Europe's Middle Ages embraced vegetarianism as part of their ascetic lifestyle, modeling themselves on Saint Jerome and Saint Geneviève. Later champions included artist Leonardo da Vinci, poet Percy Bysshe Shelley, and—as a headstrong sixteen-year-old—Benjamin Franklin.

In 1850, the American Vegetarian Society was formed by an alliance between the Reverend William Metcalfe and Sylvester Graham, the man behind the eponymous cracker. They acquired the support of Ellen G. White and the Seventh-day Adventist Church. In this latter half of the nineteenth century, vegetarianism was manifest of zealotry and associated with the cultural initiatives of anti-vivisection and temperance.

In the twentieth century, vegetarianism went mainstream. By 2002, a CNN poll would estimate that 4 percent of adults in the United States self-identified as vegetarians, and of these, 5 percent further identified themselves as vegans. The term *vegan* signifies abstinence from any animal by-product—not only meat and cheese, but wool, silk, and, for some, honey and beeswax—and was created in 1944 by the Englishman Donald Watson, who pronounced it "the beginning and end of *veg*etarian."

The rise of vegetarianism in America has corresponded with the rise of soy. Tofurkey is a legitimate Thanksgiving dish; a request for soymilk at Starbucks is as commonplace as a request for half-and-half. Though fermented soymilk has been around since the Han dynasty, soy's ascension in American cuisine can be attributed, in part, to the unlikely threesome of George Washington Carver, Henry Ford, and John Kellogg.

Dr. John Harvey Kellogg had been involved with the Seventh-day Adventists since James White (husband of Ellen) had paid a visit to the Kellogg home in 1864, when John was twelve. After receiving his medical degree from Bellevue Hospital, he became the administrator of the Adventist sanitarium and the editor of *Good Health Magazine,* in which he continually promoted a diet of fruit, nuts, and grain, no meat required.

He is often regarded as a quack nowadays, thanks to caricatures such as T. C. Boyle's novel *The Road to Wellville* and the subsequent movie it spawned. Yet in 1906, his Battle Creek Sanitarium hosted seven thousand of the country's most influential citizens (plus or minus a few neurotics). Kellogg prescribed generous consumption of water with all meals. He expressed an aversion to reliance on cow by-products, preferring milks made from almonds and hazelnuts, that would prove prescient to our understanding of the lactose intolerance that became steadily more common in the years to follow. It's a cruel irony that the cereals that bear his name brand—as trademarked by his brother, Will—have mutated into sugary bowlfuls of denatured wheat, "best" drenched in milk.

In a 1938 letter, the scientist George Washington Carver declared, "Every intelligent person interested in health, I am very certain, appreciates what Dr. Kellogg is doing. He really is my ideal." In 1911, Carver was preparing a five-course luncheon of fourteen dishes all made with peanut products (including soup, bread, creamed chicken, and dessert cookies), which he would serve to a table of the Tuskegee Institute's luminaries that included Booker T. Washington, Tuskegee's head physician, and their wives. As later enshrined in history, the meal was meant to prove the legume's value. Kellogg was the person Carver chose to send an advance copy of the menu.

Their correspondence ranged from a celebration of peanut milk to a debate over the tastiness of alfalfa salads. Kellogg feared them too bitter. "I have tried mine with several dressings," Carver wrote to him, "but I like the French dressing best. I certainly thank you for calling my attention to the lemon juice instead of the vinegar. It is delicious."

Though Carver is known for his work with peanuts and sweet potatoes, his personal tastes were far more diverse. Decades before Terra (i.e., taro) Chips became a popular boutique brand in the 1990s, he wrote to a professor at the University of Hawaii's Agricultural Experiment Station: "I grew a few Tara [sic] plants and I like them very very much. I am especially fond of the chips made from them . . . better than I do those made from the Irish potato." Since 1903 Carver had labored on using soy to create everything from ice cream to cheese to coffee to flour. In a 1936 interview, he described the soy bean as "almost, if not quite, as versatile as the peanut with its three hundred products."

This was music to Henry Ford's ears. Since 1928 he had been a student of "farm chemurgy," which sought to link farm crops to industrial products. His mission had grown particularly pointed in the wake of the Great Depression—and, as determined by the Ford Motor Company's top researchers, soy was his best prospect. At the 1934 World's Fair in Chicago, Ford had invited reporters to a fourteen-course meal (possibly in homage to Carver's earlier luncheon) in which every course consisted at least partially of soy, from soybean bread to pineapple rings with soybean cheese and soybean dressing. Not coincidentally, the very next year was when the Glidden Company in Chicago, Illinois, built the first commercial plant for industrial-grade soy proteins.

In 1934, Ford had struck up a correspondence with Carver. In March 1938, Ford toured Carver's Tuskegee lab for the first time. (Later, after declining health impaired Carver's mobility, Ford would pay to have an elevator installed on campus so he could continue his experiments.) Ford asked Carver to create a nuanced color stain—he had proposed a soy-derived mixture that mimicked cherrywood—worthy of the floor at the Powerhouse of Ford's seventy-five-thousand-acre estate in Ways Station, Georgia.

As Ford charged ahead with his efforts to manufacture a 1,400-pound car, made significantly lighter with the addition of soy plastics, Carver could not help but notice his new client's obsession. In a letter to a friend, Carver mentioned Ford was "now wearing a suit of clothes made from the soybean, so his secretary tells me." (This synthetic soybean-based silk, called Azlon, ultimately lost out to DuPont's nylon product in the commercial market.) Although they enjoyed an enduring friendship, Carver soon hit a plateau of formal involvement with Ford's vision for a soy-driven future.

"My work I endeavor to keep so that the man farthest down can profit by it," he told a South African colleague in 1940. "I am not so much interested in factories."

Ford's cars, which utilized compounds of resin and isolate

based on soy's cellulose fiber structure, proved lightweight and sturdy—Ford tested the doors with the swing of his own ax. But much to his chagrin, the panels were never 100 percent waterproof. Soy's role in the automotive industry would not be fully realized until the next century, when there was a renewed interest in biofuels.

Yet enough groundwork had been laid. Going into World War II, soy was singled out as a valued commodity. While traditional coffee beans were rationed, soy coffee, backed by Ford, flourished in popularity despite its lack of caffeine. As a high-yield, versatile crop that could enrich soil through its nitrogen fixation, soy captured the brass ring of government subsidy. By 2000, the United States produced 75 million tons of "garden" (edible) and "field" (industrial oil) soybeans.

As Michael Pollan notes in his book *In Defense of Food*, soy has become second only to corn in its prevalence in the American diet: "75 percent of the vegetable oils in your diet come from soy," he notes. "Corn contributes 554 calories a day to America's per capita food supply and soy another 257."

Soy flour is used in fast-food hamburger buns, not to mention pizza, doughnuts, and most mass-production loaves of bread. Soy protein appears in everything from hamburger meat to canned tuna to chocolate. If a child demonstrates an allergy to cow milk, soy-based infant formula is the go-to substitute available in liquid, powdered, and concentrate forms. Because of the recent positioning of edamame as a "superfood," handfuls of the immature soybean show up in everything from frozen stir-fry mixes to Applebee's salads.

When you're allergic to soy, as I am, it's a little nightmarish. In restaurants, this is what I often encounter:

Phase 1: "I have allergies I need to warn you about," I say. Waiter tenses up.

Phase 2: "Beef, dairy, egg . . ." I begin the list. Waiter noticeably relaxes. "No problem!" I hear. "We've got a variety of healthy vegetarian options."

Phase 3: I explain that actually, because of my soy allergy, I need to avoid all tofu, tempeh, and "textured vegetable protein" (the stuff of veggie burger patties). No soy mayo. No dairy-free margarine.

Phase 4: "And I'd like a carnivorous option, please. But no beef or shrimp."

Phase 5: "I'll see. I'll see what we can do." The waiter walks back to the kitchen to talk to the chef, shoulders slumped. I have managed to outfuss the *vegetarians*.

Fortunately, for now, those with IgE sensitivity to soy tend not to be as reactive as those with allergies to peanuts and shellfish. It often takes exposure to upwards of 400 milligrams of soy before an attack is induced. Dipping my sushi in a bit of soy sauce doesn't seem to bother me, and while I try to steer clear of soy oil, I can make do when I have to (which is often, since many restaurants use it exclusively in their cooking).

As a culture, we're playing with fire. For centuries Asians have included soy in their diets with little ill effect, sure. But there we're talking about primarily fermented products such as miso and *natto*, at an average of 9 grams a day. Here, we're talking about soy shakes that serve up twice that daily amount of unfermented protein in one to-go cup, complete with bendy straw. No one knows why peanut allergies have ratcheted up so rapidly in their severity. If the same happens with soy—

which, unlike corn, is already one of the "big eight" allergens in terms of its prevalence—we'll have put ourselves in a culinary chokehold.

Another troubling complication of our relationship to soy is the fact that people have a capacity to react to the allergen even without soy-sensitive IgE markers. This is part of a subset of food allergies known as oral allergy syndrome (OAS), usually found among adults with severe hay fever, in which close similarity between a food protein and pollen protein causes cross-reactivity. Essentially, your mast cells mistake one for the other. Almonds, apples, celery, and peaches are confused with alder pollen. Grass pollen has a molecular echo in melons, tomatoes, and oranges. Ragweed pairs off with banana, cantaloupe, and cucumber.

Often the full extent of the reaction is nothing more than a tingling, itching, or swelling around the lips and mouth, perhaps with gastrointestinal complications. Skinning or cooking a fruit, such as apples, may sufficiently denature the proteins to disrupt this effect. But other OAS targets, such as celery, are stubborn in their allergenicity. And the soybean? Soy does a wicked birch impression so convincing to the body that ingesting soymilk has triggered anaphylactic reactions in people sensitive to the tree pollen.

Why is soy so popular, again?

The bean is not evil. It's just a plant, one that offers complete proteins. But it has been manipulated far beyond its original forms, with even its waste products (lecithin) now marketed as all-purpose emulsifiers.

Though he was a pioneer in food science, George Washington Carver was also an advocate of farm-to-table eating. He often dined on wild mustard, turnips, and tomatoes gathered locally, using pig's feet or possum as a condiment rather than the main course. He decried those who would "make pretty plates" or value ease of preparation over nutritional value.

Long before Pollan came along with his manifesto, Carver warned us that "the science and practice of agriculture are intimate and inseparable companions, and under no circumstances should be divorced." This is not the future he had in mind.

. . .

Maybe this is jealousy talking. Maybe my resentment of King Soy is really aimed at Princess Vegan: those cute girls my sister's age, a decade younger and lither than I am, nursing their soy lattes and running in shorts that declare BROWN and UCSD across their trim posteriors.

I have never "gone" running. I have run from dogs, and I have run toward buses as they pulled away from the stop, but I don't think that counts. I do recognize the value of physical exertion, in theory. In 1999, I bought tennis shoes, as part of a summer spent trying to convince myself that I enjoyed racquetball matches at the William & Mary recreation center with my then boyfriend. The shoes' bright purple Swooshes promised a breakthrough of physical prowess. I would play! I would love it!

The whites on those shoes are still white. The laces' double-knotted bows are, I believe, vintage spring 2003.

I can't blame lack of opportunity. My father was determined to see, early on, if I would take to a sport. I remember the Saturdays when he would take me out to the fields behind various local high schools. He'd tote a big nylon sack filled with every imaginable piece of gaming equipment—aluminum bat, softball, mitt, football, soccer ball, basketball, tennis racket, two tennis balls, and, in what had to be sheer desperation, a volleyball. He pitched, caught, lobbed, set, and served, all the while looking for some raw spark of talent on my part.

I played along, happy to spend time with my dad. Every ball I hit or kicked dribbled lazily along. If there's such a thing as bunting in soccer, I am a master. I served the tennis ball short. I served the volleyball wide. After two hours, I asked, "Can we go to Long John Silver's now?"

He would have better luck when my sister came along; his principal concern over her vegetarianism was that it would not provide enough calcium and protein to sustain her not inconsiderable soccer skills. For me, between the chronic asthma and the allergies to pollen and grass, it didn't feel like I was meant to be running around outside. Sports are all about developing confidence in your body. I didn't trust mine.

With so little physical exertion, I was not the skinniest child, though I don't ever remember being teased for my weight. In middle school, the difference from one girl's figure to the next became more obvious. I hoped the pudginess of my curves were not noticeable compared to my elaborate choices of skirts, necklaces, and brooches.

In the eighth grade, while on a sleepover at my best friend's house, I pulled out one of the Mead composition notebooks she used as diaries. Melody had left the room to go talk to her mom. The diary wasn't hard to find; she kept them lined up along the headboard of her bed. I opened the marbled black-and-white cover and thumbed to the page that described our meeting on the first day of school, assigned as science partners.

The first thing she noticed about me, she had written, was my creamy, pale skin. *She is funny and a little rotund,* she had written.

Rotund?

I had spent hours picking out my outfit for that first day—the short black skirt that my mother described as "flattering," the strands of multicolored seed beads, and my one button-down shirt that, because it was draped silk, did not pucker awkwardly when I turned to the side to eye my burgeoning bustline. The shirt was a shade that the saleswoman at the Limited called "cinnamon," and I called "orange."

I blushed. *I must have looked like the Great Pumpkin,* I thought. The diary was back on the shelf by the time Melody returned to the room, but the damage was done to my self-esteem.

My mother, then in her early forties, was and is a strikingly beautiful woman—a onetime Cherry Blossom Princess for the state of Illinois (though, as her mother insists, "it was much more about academics back then")—who didn't keep much junk food in the house. Even if she had chocolate syrup and ice cream around, I couldn't have eaten them because of my milk allergy. Where were these extra pounds coming from?

It would take another decade for me to recognize that the problem rested on minor dietary choices (Pringles over pretzels, skin-on versus skinless chicken) exacerbated by a major case of overeating. If my mother made Rice Krispies treats in the morning, I'd have eaten half the pan by 4 p.m. I once ate an entire pack of chicken wings in two hours.

It was not that my parents had ever forced me into the clean-plate club; even a slightly "off" feeling was grounds to abandon a meal. Yet when we found a Sandra-friendly food, particularly when traveling or being hosted by others, I was encouraged to feed until I was absolutely, 100 percent full. And then just a little more.

I remember breakfasts of not one, not two, but four McDonald's hash browns, with 36 grams of fat—80 percent of my entire recommended fat intake for the day. We knew it wasn't healthy. But we also knew they'd stop making those patties at 10:30 a.m. And no one knew how long it would be before I found a safe harbor to eat lunch.

Somewhere along the way my mind stopped connecting a satiated stomach with any instinct to stop eating. I will eat until an available dish is exhausted. In the case of a whole roast chicken, that means after I've used my little finger to tease the last of the moist meat from the crevices around the scapula. In the case of a trip to Five Guys, that means every last fry crumb in the bag. In the case of a party at my house, that means using every leftover slice of rosemary bread to swipe up all the remaining garlic hummus, long past the hour when dip has started to dry and flake off the edges of its plastic tub.

In the last few years, I have forged an uneasy truce with my appetite. I am learning to cook, and occasionally (particularly with company), I'll sit down with an actual meal: turkey with quinoa and curried root vegetables, or tomatillo chicken with black beans and guacamole. But more often, accepting my instinct to gorge, I settle for striking a nutritional balance over multiple meals, rather than on any one plate.

"What *do* you eat?" people usually ask upon first hearing of my allergies.

"Plenty of things," I answer. "Couscous, chickpeas, almonds, fish, apples, oatmeal, spinach, wild rice, chicken, broccoli . . ."

All true. I just don't admit that—outside of restaurants and other special occasions—it will probably be only one or two of those foods at any given time, with the barest of dressing or sauce, heaped in a bowl intended for serving to a table of four.

I suspect that the regimen associated with food allergies elicits disordered eating patterns for many people. But it's hard to find a commiserative community. In public we fixate on the opposite dynamic, in which those with disordered eating patterns use food allergies to justify their behaviors. Anorexics claim they have gone vegetarian. Bulimics chalk up gastric distress to "some kind of intolerance." Celebrities pass on bread during an interview, then assure the media that it's not that they don't eat carbs—it's that they're allergic to wheat.

A 2010 article in the Daily Beast touted "The New Star Diet Craze":

"Gluten-free" living was, for years, about as sexy as living with diabetes, a conversation-killer and a dinner-party bummer. . . . Despite all this, or perhaps because of it, a gluten-free diet has become synonymous with enlightened eating, an intellectual aesthetic with its own raft of studies and its own celebrity cache. In fact, Hollywood is suddenly overrun with gluten allergies. Jenny McCarthy is convinced it contributed to her son's autism. Gwyneth Paltrow blames it for her extra "holiday" pounds. The View's Elisabeth Hasselbeck says it caused her years of chronic pain. And they all gush with near-religious fervor about their restful nights, their clear skin, their freedom from seasonal allergies, and the general *joie de vivre* their wheat-free regimens bring.

Does anyone else see the weird logical leap made here? An article that cites three celebrities who have given up wheat for reasons *other* than food allergies (Hasselbeck has celiac disease) announces Hollywood is "suddenly overrun with gluten allergies." In other words, allergies are something you claim for the sake of being contrarian ("Despite all this, or perhaps *because of it*") or justifying an extreme diet; they are a stylish look, like cinched belts or faux-hawks, you can don for one fashion season and ditch the next.

In 2007, pop star Jessica Simpson announced to an interviewer for *Elle* magazine that the minor internal bleeding she experienced while filming *Employee of the Month* was explained when "doctors found the presence of the little bugger thought to cause ulcers." Somehow further (though unsubstantiated) discomfort led to a diagnosis of allergy to "cheese, wheat, tomatoes, hot peppers, coffee, corn, and chocolate."

Huh. If the "little bugger" of *H. pylori* bacterium was a problem, then their mention is a bit of a red herring—diet is not a key cause for peptic ulcers, though a bland diet is recommended during recovery. More relevant may have been the fact that coming off 2005's *The Dukes of Hazzard*, this was the skinniest stretch in Simpson's adult career. All of her newfound allergens happened to coincide with many of the foods one would embargo to maintain a size-2 figure.

I can't remember allergies mentioned in a single episode of *Newlyweds: Nick and Jessica* (I admit I watched far too many), though there were plenty of eating scenes. As commentators at the Consumerist website were quick to point out, her sensitivity to cheese, wheat, and tomatoes hadn't kept her from signing on as Pizza Hut's spokeswoman. Based on my milk allergy alone, no amount of money could make me pose with a slice of pie within an arm's reach of my face. Hives and vomiting don't make for a pretty commercial.

It's hard to be sure where the truth lies when someone like the actor Billy Bob Thornton opens up about having allergies to wheat, shellfish, and dairy—as well as obsessive-compulsive disorder and past anorexia. The celebrity allergies I find most credible are linked to public incidents—as when the singer Kelis had to be rushed to a Zurich hospital after being exposed to nuts while on tour—or are attributed to stars with no rabid fan base. No one is craving trivia about comic Ray Romano so they can scribble *peanuts* under the "Dislikes" column of his *Tiger Beat* poster.

I do not live or die by whether Jessica Simpson can secretly enjoy the occasional morning coffee and Danish. This is no more my business than was my sister's decision to become a vegetarian. But that's the thing about body politics; it's impossible not to have a gut take on these issues, and it's always rooted in the bias of your own skin and bones.

Almost ten years into her decision, Christina is still a vegetarian. Even if she changes her mind tomorrow, it will have been no mere indulgence or whim. What once seemed like an older sister's wisdom, I now recognize was my stubborn resistance to admitting she was old enough to make her own choices. I'd like to think I'd not make that mistake again. But allergies tangle the ties that bind us, whether bloodlines or food chains.

CHAPTER SIX

Gilding the Gouda

Luring the average American into becoming a "foodie" is now a multibillion-dollar industry. I have taken the bait, after years of eating in a manner that was at best ascetic and at worst disordered. There is no other explanation for my decision to wake up at eight on a Saturday morning, catch a taxi downtown, and find myself at an event populated by men like Mike. Mike, whose chest hair froths beyond the top button of his Hawaiian shirt. Mike, who will be handling our loin today.

"That's good," Giada De Laurentiis says. She moves her hands in small demonstrative circles, encouraging him to massage salt and pepper all over the pork's surface. While the rest of the undercaffeinated audience blinks owlishly from our seats, Mike has jumped up to share the stage with De Laurentiis, host of the show *Everyday Italian.* Confident and beaming, in his midfifties, he knows his way around a loin. I'm transfixed by the feisty tuft of silver chest hair above the collar of his dark shirt. Does he comb it out each morning?

A large crowd has settled into the 2,700 seats that occupy one section of one room in the gargantuan Walter E. Washington Convention Center. This is the kickoff cooking demonstration of the fourth annual Metropolitan Cooking & Entertaining Show. There will be standing room only for Paula Deen and Guy Fieri later this afternoon. But we have come to watch Giada "because," as my friend Amy puts it, "she is so beautiful."

Giada is a slim-hipped waif, dressed in clingy layers of gray silk fit for a ballet dancer. A black scarf loops loosely around her neck, lending bulky modesty to an otherwise bare collarbone. Her amber hair sits in a high bun on top of her head. On me, the style would look like junior-year homecoming. On her, it looks perfect.

Because Mike is so gung ho in his meat prep, Giada is free to step to the front of the stage and take a round of questions. Question one is "How do you stay so thin?"

"You can eat anything," she says, "if you eat it in moderation." She will claim this three more times during the course of the hour.

Our host's petite beauty emphasizes the surreal, dollhouse efficiency of the cooking setup that surrounds her. It's as if the producers chopped a kitchen in half: a gleaming fridge, two ovens, a stovetop, a sink with running water, a food processor, and a blender, all wired and ready to go in a "room" with only one wall. Whatever it costs, the organizers can afford it; this convention has just been named one of the fifty fastest-growing tradeshows in the country.

I missed the first wave of Food Network enthusiasm in the midnineties, when housewives flocked to Emeril Lagasse's dynamic broadcasts. A second wave of cooking-show love crested around 2002, washing over my fellow graduate students and other underemployed twentysomethings. Friends debated Mario Batali versus Bobby Flay, but I stayed out of it. My knowledge of cooking shows consisted of dim childhood memories of whatever came on PBS after *Sesame Street:* Julia Child, *The Frugal Gourmet*, *Louisiana Cookin'* with Justin Wilson—all of whom worshipped at the altar of butter, cream, and fat, or, as Graham Kerr of *The Galloping Gourmet* called it, "hedonism in a hurry." Even Martin Yan of *Yan Can Cook* was always throwing a little chopped egg into the stir-fry. Why taunt myself?

Then came Rachael Ray. Love her or hate her, Ray raised the profile of extra-virgin olive oil ("EVOO") right as a number of health studies began touting the benefits of the Mediterranean diet. Even before catching her show, I'd noticed her impact in restaurants. Turning down salad dressing, which used to puzzle waiters, now solicited a cheery if initially indecipherable "Eee-veedoubleoh, then?" The acronym became so pervasive that it was indexed by *The Oxford American College Dictionary* in 2007.

So here I am on a Saturday morning, another convert. Giada twists the cap off the big green bottle of oil, readying her vinaigrette. She charges Mike, his hands already slick, with dropping any pungent ingredients into the blender. He asks if he needs gloves.

"No, you don't need gloves," Giada says. Then she reconsiders. "Unless you do. Are you allergic to garlic?"

Mike shakes his head and goes to work. This is a new era;

Julia Child never asked about food allergies. As Giada loads the raw tenderloin into the oven and—the magic of television—pulls it out, fully cooked, from the other oven, I sigh in satisfaction with the rest of the audience. Not only could I make this meal, I could actually eat it.

"Next up, rigatoni with shrimp," Giada says. *Damn.* This will not be a recipe I can use. She walks over to the shiny stunt fridge and opens the door with a flourish to reveal . . . an empty shelf.

"The shrimp are not in the fridge," she announces, looking offstage for help. The young crewman shrugs. This is the peril of being the first demo of the day. "We are improvising!" Giada says. "No shrimp!"

Her next audience assistant is Linda, a twentysomething woman in thick-rimmed glasses and an olive green cardigan. Linda swears she is the biggest fan ever.

"Do you cook?" Giada asks.

"I clean vegetables," Linda replies.

"What about pasta?"

"I clean vegetables," Linda says again, firmly.

With no shellfish handy, Giada has decided to fix rigatoni with butternut squash. The squash is already peeled and diced, meaning there are no vegetables to clean. Linda tenses her shoulders at this news. Giada is held captive behind the counter, guiding her step by step, while the lineup of audience members with questions grows longer.

Giada hands Linda the box of pasta. Linda dumps it in.

Giada asks her to grind the pepper. Linda turns the knob over and over, robotic, until our host places a hand on her arm to stop her.

"Otherwise," she says, "we'll be serving a plate of pepper with pasta, not pasta with pepper."

Giada tells Linda to cut some basil. When she picks up the correct herb, one of only two bunches on the counter, Giada cheers, "Good for you!"

The pace is tedious, but at least it is easy to follow. I could re-create this later. Then, as the squash is sautéing, a carton of milk materializes in Giada's hand. Where did that come from? And why is she—*Noooo!*

"You see how it's coming together?" she asks Linda, pointing her spoon into the pot. "Loosening up, becoming nice and creamy?"

Giada picks up a big, firm triangle of cheese and a long, thin grater. "Lots of Parmesan," she says, grating it in. "Then grill the shrimp and throw 'em on."

This often happens when I watch cooking shows. I'll sit patiently, taking notes for fifteen minutes, only to realize some clutch ingredient renders the whole recipe useless to me. My salt-water pasta lacks creaminess. It will always lack creaminess. I am doomed to a life of lackluster, shrimp-less pasta.

Giada, on the other hand, lives with a gourmet's passion. She clasps her hands to her chest and swoons at the mention of squash blossom fritters. A bona fide swoon; her body mic booms. She lights up when an audience member asks how to fix *struffoli,* telling him to lift the deep-fried dough out the moment the honey begins to crystallize, rhapsodizing that it is a favorite treat in her hometown.

Did I mention how perfectly thin she is?

The dessert is something involving ricotta and crumbles of biscotti, neither of which I can eat. The volunteer assistants have been increasingly starstruck and decreasingly helpful, and by this point the stage is crowded with the next generation of foodies: five girls ages ten to twelve, a five-year-old whose eyes barely clear the demonstration counter, a pregnant woman who introduces her protruding belly as "Megan," and one other extremely sheepish-looking grown-up.

As Giada spoons cheese into a food processor, I have no useful reference point for how this would or could taste. Maybe this is the true definition of pornography—being invited to take satisfaction in images devoid of larger meaning. My mind wanders back to college days, when one of my guy friends would pop into another's dorm room and announce, "I got a Shakira video off Napster." I loved that these guys had broadened their musical horizons to include Latin girl-pop. Then I realized they were watching Shakira with the sound turned off.

Up onstage, in response to repeated pulses of the blades, the espresso powder blending into the ricotta makes for a sexy, sultry brown cream. But it's an empty pleasure for me. There's no future in it. I feel an urge to shower.

Our hour with Giada is up. She thanks us and retreats backstage. Amy and I follow the crowd toward row after row of sponsor displays and vendor tables, each offering a little taste of something. It's dizzying: FunniBonz Barbeque, BelGioioso Cheese, Belmont Peanuts, Pestos with Panache, Red Rocker Candy, McNulty's Chutney.

Cutting a wide berth around the cheese, I focus on the possibilities. I've never seen so many salsas. Each proprietor sizes you up as you pass the table. Are you a potential sale? Sample mooch? Food journalist? They don't appreciate me spinning jars around to examine labels. I am messing with their display.

For every dip or sauce I decide I can try, there's the consequent challenge of getting it to my mouth. The only serving utensils are in the form of unmarked chips and pretzels. I have to be careful. A pretzel used to consist of flour, yeast, and salt, but now even mainstream varieties use buttermilk. Some tortilla chips use a lime flavor that is bound with a milk derivative.

"May I ask what kind of chips these are?" I ask one seller, hoping he'll produce a bag I can check for ingredients.

"The cheap kind," he says. "What do you want to know about my salsa?"

I'm impeding the flow of valuable traffic. Most of these vendors don't have national shelf presence; they rely on Internet sales, bulk orders, and the hope that some enthused blogger will set their product on the path to viral popularity. As entrepreneurs, they know that lack of everyday access is a deal breaker for many customers. People who smile over a free sample will ultimately choose a cheap Trader Joe's variation or something they can get delivered to their house by Peapod.

Many will choose those routes. Not all. Not the foodies, and not the parents of food-allergic children, for whom stalking brands across time and distance is everyday housekeeping. When Duncan Hines pulled the one Sandra-friendly, store-bought oatmeal raisin cookie from the shelves of local grocery stores, my mother made a special deal with the distributor to buy cookies by the case until the manufacturer's supply ran out. We became proselytizers, giving a pack to any parents who had a house I might visit to play with their kids.

Somewhere in between the fifteenth spicy salsa and the

twentieth hot sauce, I begin to feel tingly, with what is either a glimmer of hope or an overdose of capsaicin. What I'm thinking is, what makes someone a foodie? A pickiness toward brands; an obsession over provenance; a curiosity about cooking technique? What are traits common to a food-allergic adult? All the same ones. Maybe my genetics haven't cursed me to a lifetime of boring meals. Maybe they have made me a natural-born foodie.

I see a large crowd huddled around a demonstration, and walk over to find Carla Hall, of cable television fame, making peanut soup. Hall is a longtime Washingtonian who teaches at CulinAerie, one of D.C.'s newer catering service/cooking school ventures. She became a fan favorite during the fifth season of Bravo's *Top Chef* in part because of her positive attitude ("cook with love"), and in part because of her refusal to fix anything that didn't truly nourish the body.

Hall's competition highlight, for me, was when contestants were asked to serve a cocktail pairing for their food. A nondrinker herself, the "chef-testant" didn't compromise her ethics by using spirits. She didn't fake it with a mocktail masking the lack of alcohol. Instead, she made a cranberry and ginger spritzer based on key lime soda, a drink not trying to be anything other than what it was—delicious.

Now she is ladling out tastes of the soup to the hungry crowd. Someone asks about avoiding the calories of heavy cream, and Hall mentions using tofu to thicken the consistency of her broth. An older man asks if she ever wants to open her own restaurant, and she says no. I ask if CulinAerie has ever thought about offering classes for those with food allergies. She looks at me.

"I think it's a really good idea. The class would be all about substitutions, right? If you have milk, *use this*. If you can't eat peanuts, *use this*."

I should be happy at her enthusiasm, but my heart sinks. All about substitutions? There are so many worthy dishes. She could have said that one could program a gourmet cooking class without ever needing to use (or substitute for) milk, peanuts, eggs, or wheat. Instead she articulated the allergen-centric mentality I am trying to shake. The one that whispers, *You'll never really be one of us.*

An assistant tries to hand me a Dixie cup of Carla's soup, but I shake my head. I didn't catch the ingredients. Knowing it was "cooked with love" doesn't quite cover it.

· · ·

I grew up a conservative eater, slow to expand my palate. Even though I knew to ask for olive oil in restaurants, it wasn't until I was twenty years old, standing at a salad bar and looking down at a bin of chopped black olives, that I thought, *Oh. I bet I can eat those, too.* I avoided eggplant for years, not because I'd had reactions to other nightshade plants but because the echo of *egg* made me nervous. Certain foods, like lobster, were too intimidating to fix at home and too expensive to test in public. I came to appreciate repetition and dishes in which the simplicity is its own aesthetic.

A few years ago, I was at a friend's party and complaining about fusion cuisine. The fusion trend means there is always some nouveau element, such as pesto foam or a garnish of chili-chocolate shavings, that renders a dish deadly in a way

I could not have anticipated from the menu description. I hate taking one look at a plate and sending it back. It's a waste of their food and of my time.

But, oh, sushi! My rant gradually turned into an ode to sushi. Fresh fish, combined in elegant ways according to traditional assembly techniques. No random slices of honeydew. No hoity-toity vinaigrettes. Sushi is safe. Sushi is sacred.

The boyfriend of the hostess, who happened to be the managing editor of a local monthly magazine, proposed that I write a roundup of Washington's sushi joints. My article included instructions on how to handle *nigiri* with chopsticks, orgasmic praise of high-grade salmon sashimi, and an extreme close-up of seaweed salad—tangled and dripping with sesame oil—that would have been at home in an issue of *Penthouse*. Readers responded, and the magazine offered me a regular gig as a reviewer.

It was then I discovered that despite two decades of caution, I loved food. I loved writing about culinary trivia. I relished knowing that the mango was related to the cashew, which was related to the pistachio, facts gathered as part of a know-thy-enemy strategy. I could ask about the base of a Vietnamese *pho* (beef broth? shrimp? vegetable?) not as an allergic obsessive but as a Food Writer.

I invited my family to accompany me on a few "research" meals in the city, relying on their impressions to complement my own. After years of altering her orders so that I could have a taste, my mother welcomed the task of ordering exactly what I *couldn't* have. She was my go-to expert on coconut-crusted shrimp.

My father, perhaps waxing nostalgic for his days in the

army's Psychological Operations unit, seemed to most relish the covert aspect of reviewing. Yet he didn't exactly play it cool; he always made sure to introduce himself to the house manager using his (and my) last name. After one dinner of jerk chicken and fried plantains, he raved about the coffee. A Caribbean import, he could tell. He insisted we find out the blend's name in case I wanted to work it into the review.

The waiter returned shortly. "Maxwell House, sir! Fresh made."

Much as I enjoyed the gig, I was not destined to be the next Ruth Reichl. The limitations of my abilities became increasingly apparent. I was assigned to review an Italian restaurant specializing in pizza, which I would report in my review served thin crusts "crisped to perfection." I claimed "to perfection" based on my lunch date liking her Pizza Margherita. She said the mozzarella was "tasty," which I dutifully recorded.

Tasty. That was all I had to go on. My dish was dry pasta— hold the cheese, hold the chorizo, hold the meat sauce. Definitely not the house specialty. How could I judge them based on that? This wasn't how the chef had designed his flavor profile. This was how I'd forced them to fix it.

My reviews became regurgitated ingredient lists, prettied up with adjectives. Then my editor suggested that I review a new French restaurant. I tried to picture a Gallic meal without butter or cheese or beef, and I told them the jig was up. In two short years, my critical reign had come and gone.

Even the chefs can find themselves on the wrong side of an allergy-unfriendly menu. In a 2009 piece for *The Atlantic*, Ming Tsai—a Chinese-American chef, James Beard Foundation Award–winner, and host of public television's *Simply Ming*—

described being turned away from a Massachusetts restaurant based on his five-year-old son's allergies. Before being seated, Tsai asked to speak to a manager and warned him of his son's severe sensitivities to peanuts, tree nuts, wheat, soy, dairy, egg, and shellfish.

"Instead of being greeted with a can-do attitude or any amount of graciousness," Tsai recounts, "I was literally told 'We'd prefer not to serve you.'"

Tsai, now a spokesperson for the Food Allergy and Anaphylaxis Network, resolved to change the attitudes of restaurateurs in his home state. At his restaurant Blue Ginger, opened in Wellesley in 1998, Tsai developed a "Food Allergy Reference Book." This three-ring binder lists the ingredients of every menu item to provide efficient, reliable answers to queries. No more saying, as I have heard so often, "We don't know what's in the soup because the chef is gone for the night."

From washing dishes to de-croutoning salads to shaking out linen napkins, every aspect of Blue Ginger's service has been refined to head off cross-contamination. Tsai emphasizes that the key to creating a safe kitchen is good (and no-cost) technique, not pricey substitutions. He asks his prep chefs to keep ingredients as separate as possible for as long as possible, a habit already somewhat ingrained in kitchen culture.

"Everyone knows to wash their board and knife thoroughly, if not change out their board entirely, after working with raw chicken because of the risk of salmonella," Tsai wrote in his article. "At Blue Ginger, every ingredient is raw chicken."

Thanks in part to lobbying by Tsai and FAAN, in 2009, Massachusetts passed the Food Allergy Awareness Act (Senate Bill 2701). This bill requires all restaurants to display an allergen awareness poster in the kitchen that details the "big eight" allergens, describes reaction symptoms, and prescribes response protocol. Restaurants must request on their menus that customers inform servers of their allergies before ordering. (This provides some liability protection to the vendors as well.) They must train managers about responding to those with allergy concerns, using a video developed through a partnership with FAAN and the Massachusetts Restaurant Association.

A restaurant that complies with these standards and, in addition, voluntarily develops its own "Food Allergy Reference Book," is eligible for a "food-allergy friendly" designation from the Massachusetts Department of Public Health.

Legislations comparable to parts or all of these guidelines have also been introduced in Minnesota, New York, Connecticut, and Pennsylvania. But even where the government has not gotten involved, there is rising awareness of the need for a coordinated response to those with allergies. The National Restaurant Association provides its membership with a free booklet, "Welcoming Guests with Food Allergies," that articulates some of the delicate cultural issues I've dealt with firsthand. If you've ever identified yourself as a customer with allergies, know that:

Yes, they've been told to give you a knowledgeable, senior contact person for your order. So if you suddenly have a new waiter, it's not some form of rejection.

Yes, they've been told they must discard any accidentally tainted plate and start from scratch. If you suspect this has not happened, you have a right to insist on it. (None of this brushing Parmesan from the rim of the spaghetti plate and serving it back to me. Vivace in Charlottesville, that's right, I'm looking at you.)

Yes, the ultimate decision on what is "safe" belongs to the customer. If your gut says that the dish they bring out will make you sick—whether because of a botched order or an untrustworthy server—you can politely decline, you should not be billed, and you should not feel guilty.

This last guideline makes me regret all the "absolutely nondairy" sorbets I've been bullied into trying for dessert. I could have saved a lot of time, pain, and money if I'd just given myself permission to say, "Sorry, I don't think that's going to work, after all," at the sight of a stray swirl of another flavor.

The Culinary Institute of America (CIA), in partnership with the National Peanut Board, offers even more extensive guidance through its website. They are trying to reach the chefs of the future as well as the restaurants of today. Frankly, the industry needs the help. It's a little terrifying to see a survey of one hundred dining establishments, conducted by the Jaffe Food Allergy Institute at Mount Sinai School of Medicine, in which 24 percent believes "a small amount is safe" and 35 percent believe fryer heat destroys allergens. For me, the latter is particularly troubling when it comes to menus that offer deep-fried shrimp or fried mozzarella sticks alongside French fries.

The CIA site breaks it down, rule by rule: Do not reuse pasta water that was used to cook cheese-filled gnocchi. Do not reuse a cutting board that hosted Asiago bread. Know that cold cuts of mortadella sausage carry traces of nuts, and that fake crab often contains fish and egg. Don't forget the cheese hidden in a pesto that may have been made earlier in the day.

Wheat shows up in soy sauce, bouillon cubes, and ice cream. If someone orders chicken and is allergic to beef, check before using the same grill surface.

One CIA webpage is devoted to easy variations on proteins and spreads. Adapting recipes for allergies is presented not as a compromise of one's techniques but as a further dimension of knowing one's way around the kitchen. Anyone can hold the tofu on a dish for someone allergic to soy. A superior chef might know his options well enough to offer cubes of *paneer* (pressed Indian cheese) instead. Or, in my case, a chef might offer to substitute for something creamy by using a base of pureed avocado.

Safety is a right, not a luxury, though sometimes the phrasing of well-meaning restaurateurs conflates the two. I was thrilled when the innovative Spanish chef José Andrés's ThinkFoodGroup announced menus designed for those with allergies. That said, I had to giggle at their come-hither line on behalf of Café Atlántico.

"The tantalizing *Sandwich de Salmón con Malagueta*, an entrée of seared salmon with salmon salad, cucumber and mixed chips is a great choice for those allergic to dairy, soy, peanuts and tree nuts," the media release promised. Never has someone attempted to make accommodation sound so seductive.

"Oyamel's tortillas are made with corn, the ideal choice for guests avoiding wheat or gluten. Oyamel offers nine different taco options from *Tacos de Chapulines*, the legendary specialty from Oaxaca of sautéed grasshoppers, to *Carnitas con salsa de tomatillo*, confit of baby pig with green tomatillo sauce."

Finally! Grasshoppers and confit of baby pig for the rest of us. I had dreamed this day would come.

Pricey boutique entrées are one thing. What about chain restaurants? Fast food? Although sensitivity to other allergies is still developing, I've found gluten-free menus everywhere from Maggiano's Little Italy to Red Robin to Wendy's to P.F. Chang's China Bistro. At every price point, restaurants are realizing a safe customer is a repeat customer. Even Uno Chicago Grill has come up with not one but two gluten-free pizza choices.

One collaboration between the food-allergic and restaurant communities has been taking place in New York City, where "Allergic Girl" Sloane Miller has been organizing her "Worry-Free Dinner" series and membership group since 2008. Partnering with prominent venues such as Tom Colicchio's Craftbar, Miller has coordinated multicourse menus specific to particular food allergies—meaning that for a night, an entire restaurant might become peanut or dairy free. These events double as opportunities to network with other food-allergic folks and to learn Miller's tips on how to better communicate your allergy-based needs to those in the restaurant industry. For example, don't order something "plain," which is subject to interpretation by your server. Order it "only"; i.e., "Only grilled chicken and lettuce, please."

As encouraging as these breakthroughs in eating out are, to focus on them is to dance around a personal reality. I'm no longer the teenager looking for a safe place to snack with friends at the mall. I'm no longer a twentysomething with scads of disposable income. I'm at a point when I want to serve food, on my own table, rather than be served by a waiter. I want to cook.

For years I dated a man named Adam, who I had first met in the Jefferson Society at UVA. Before we moved in together, back when I lived with a roommate who monopolized the kitchen, Adam and I would go out for brunch. We would straggle the eight blocks from my place down to the Luna Grill and Diner, where our usual grizzled waitress would bring us coffee and then ask, "You set for now? I'm stepping out for a cigarette." Adam would order waffles or pancakes, slathered in butter, or eggs, folded with cheese, and I would get cinnamon-raisin oatmeal with a side of bacon.

I don't miss paying four dollars for bacon or eight dollars for oatmeal, but I miss that ritual of brunch. That said, eggs? Waffles? Pancakes? I'll never be someone who can whip up a proper brunch at home. My allergies forbid it.

Or do they?

. . .

"Honey, I need you to do me a big favor," I told Adam, walking toward his desk. "I'll pay for the whole thing."

He rolled his chair back and looked up at me with alarm. "What?"

"Do this brunch thing with me. A cooking class."

"Oh." His eyes returned to the laptop screen, where he was toggling back and forth between various Xbox help-boards for Call of Duty 4: Modern Warfare. "Sure. I thought it was going to be something a lot weirder than that."

It seemed pretty weird to me. Brunch is merciless for someone allergic to eggs, dairy, melon, and sausage. That was why I'd chosen it. Carla Hall's words had gotten under my skin, and I wanted to see how far I could get in a "normal" gourmet cooking class. No substitutes. No accommodations.

The Sunday seminar was advertised for couples, but I explained to Adam that his job was to stand by and let me do all the hands-on work. If I started to react, he should step in and take over—I didn't want to cause a scene. But the point was to prove that I could, as an adult at the age of twenty-nine, manage one little brunch all by myself.

A few weeks later, we made our way through December sleet to CulinAerie's sleek storefront in Northwest D.C. Five place settings were laid out, one per couple, complete with our own burner, mixing bowls, and spatulas. Adam sat down gratefully with a hot mug of coffee while I stayed on my feet, sizing up the field of battle.

Powdered ingredients had been premeasured and nestled next to a couple of eggs, scallions, and a small pile of shiitake mushrooms. I picked up an egg, feeling its cool heft. I eyed the meek squares of anonymous chocolate and the half cup of milk, which looked like glue in its little plastic cup. I did not touch them.

The chef, who seemed to be about our age, welcomed us. She introduced her white-aproned helpers, volunteers who soaked up the recipes for free in return for offering us help, whisking away food scraps and dirty dishes, and pouring mimosas. *Kitchen elves*, I thought, a label I would not be able to shake for the next two hours.

The advertisement for the class had listed the lineup of dishes: prosciutto and fruit, muffins, veggie frittata, and chocolate mousse. The mousse scared me, but I figured preparing the other three dishes first would build my confidence to the point of taking on milk chocolate, egg, and cream all at once.

"Now," the instructor announced. "The mousse will need

an hour to chill before serving. So let's get that assembled, first thing, and into the fridge."

As she starts talking about melting the chocolate in the double boiler, separating the egg whites, and whipping the cream, a low-grade buzz of panic rose in my ears. I stared down into my coffee, then yanked my gaze back to the front of the room, afraid I was missing something. One of the elves approached.

"Hazelnut liqueur?" she offered.

"Yes," I said gratefully.

She tipped it into the bowl. Oh. She meant for flavoring the mousse.

"What do you want me to do?" Adam asked.

"Nothing," I said. "I'm going to separate this egg."

"Are you sure? The white's gonna go everywhere."

I glared at him, then tapped the egg against the edge of the bowl. I could do this. A hairline crack formed. The second tap did nothing. I wondered if the egg would explode in my hand if I tapped harder—fearing not so much an allergic reaction as proof of my ineptitude.

I dug my thumbnail into the crack and pulled the shell apart in my hands, cupping the yolk in my palm while the rest drained down into the bowl, then hurled the yolk into the trash and bolted for the sink. I lathered and scrubbed my palms twice over. While I was slaving over a single egg, the couple next to us had already set up their Cuisinart and whipped their whites.

Adam hunched over our finicky burner, working with an elf to hook up the butane canister. The logistics of the prep were designed for four hands, and we were already behind. I decided he could take care of anything mechanical, pushing a button or turning a dial. We muddled our way through the mousse, finally scooping the mixture into two triangular cocktail tumblers that we shoved into the refrigerator. One dish down.

"Since we've already got the mixers out," said the chef, "we'll make cinnamon-sugar muffins next." More eggs. I raised my hand to request a mimosa.

We were the novices in the room. While others had been slathering decorative curves into the tops of their mousses with a spoon, Adam had been piling ours up like a kid with a sand bucket and a shovel. I tried to grate fresh nutmug into the flour and instead dropped the whole thing in, scattering the cinnamon as I tried to fish it out by hand. As we coaxed the muffin mixture into baking cups, an elf darted in to wipe away drips of batter.

"Or else it will burn," she explained.

"No, no, that's how I like my muffins," Adam told her. "That's my trademark technique." He always had a knack for using hyperbole to escape embarrassment. "This is when I add the pork," he said.

I get lucky with the fruit. "This is usually done with melon," acknowledged the instructor. "But I hate melon." We used grapes and slices of pear instead. For the first time all morning I could unabashedly work the food with my hands—peeling the pear, piercing each grape, stretching and folding the prosciutto with my fingertips so that it formed a wave undulating up the skewer.

"Those look really good," Adam hinted. I gave him one but was otherwise greedy, eating the skewers as fast as I could make them. It was past noon and all I'd had were mimosas. Adam contented himself with wolfing down some very lopsided but (so he claimed) tasty muffins.

"I can't believe they were done so fast," he said. "I can't believe I baked something. Kind of."

All around us, couples were relaxed and chatting. This was what I've always envied about gourmet eating—how a meal can stretch into hours. The lazy pace is the goal, the preparation a kind of appetizer foreplay. I wish I could make a bowl of oatmeal last this long, or look this sexy.

"Are you ready for the frittata?" the chef asked.

I was. I ran my knife through the fleshy shiitakes, stripped and diced the ginger. I skipped the garlic, though I have always admired how a clove crushes and splits under the flat of a blade. But I knew that garlic gave Adam headaches. I reached for scallions.

"Actually, can you skip those, too?" Adam asked. "I don't like them."

I wanted to say no—knife work was one of the few things I'd been good at this morning—but it was a petty point. His tongue would be the only judge of this frittata when it was done. After the skillet had been loaded into the oven, I realized there was salt and pepper at our workstation, waiting. I looked at Adam.

"Did we use salt? In anything?"

He shook his head. No difference. After it emerged from the oven and cooled, the whole frittata disappeared from his plate in thirty seconds and five bites.

Spotting my spotless knife and fork, a passing elf asked, "Did you have your frittata yet?"

"Someone stole it," Adam said, tapping his fork and knife on the counter. "I demand another."

We'd reached dessert, the mousses having set. The instructor doled out mint leaves for a garnish and suggested that those who had used the hazelnut liqueur add a spoonful of chopped hazelnuts on top as well.

"To warn people there's an unexpected ingredient," she said. "In case they have a nut allergy." I smiled. Of all this dish's ingredients, the hazelnuts were the one thing that *wouldn't* kill me.

All that was left to do was top off the mousse with fresh-whipped cream. I gripped the shallow little bowl in one hand and the whisk in the other, trying to pitch the chilled cream at an efficient angle for beating. I began to swish the whisk frantically, careful to keep each slosh of liquid shy of the bowl's lip, until my wrist started to hurt. It wouldn't take shape. I tried again. Nothing. The cream was starting to warm up, at which point it would be too late for it to set properly. So close, and yet so far.

Adam gently took the bowl from me and switched the whisk back and forth with a rapid beat. His hand and arm became spattered in white as the cream first aerated, then foamed. "You have to really get into it and take a risk," he said. "That doesn't work for someone like you."

At least, this is what I heard him say. Later I would figure out that what he actually said was "flick your wrist," not "take a risk." But my hurt ego heard what it wanted to hear: judgment. I didn't have the right stuff.

I stepped away from our cooking station. Walking over to a bank of windows, I noticed that a birthday party of ten- and eleven-year-olds had filed into the adjoining room. Cooking parties are now popular among preteens. I'm glad this wasn't the case when I was a kid. I can remember only one party that involved making something—pasta, from scratch. We had all been given the party favors of aprons, and for step one, I had made my little volcano of flour along with everyone else. Then they got the eggs out, and I had to stand back for step two. And step three. And steps four through six.

There was something odd about this CulinAerie birthday party. In addition to the usual moms, there were men stationed every ten feet, their alert postures at odds with their casual button-downs. I overheard one of the other students identify them as Secret Service. *Obama.* Apparently, a daughter of President Obama was among the party guests. Jolted out of my self-pity by this brush with celebrity, I returned to tell Adam.

The cream was now fully whipped. He was so proud. And as I watched him dollop it on our mousse, it occurred to me that I'd had this all wrong. My original plan—to make Adam stand by, passive, while I fixed everything on my own—would have been a victory, technically. But this wasn't really about skewering prosciutto instead of eating it straight from the package or learning how to give eggs an Asian flavor profile.

A gourmet glorifies food as a gesture of love, whether love for the self—eating Lean Cuisine off the good china—or love for the person sitting on the other side of the table. This was the person on the other side of my table. And he really didn't want to stand back and watch me kill myself over a mousse.

"Looks good," I said as Adam took his first bite. We were trying to build a nest in those years. It didn't matter which one of us broke the eggs.

CHAPTER SEVEN

Kiss of Death

Kiss of death for nut allergy girl," proclaimed the headline in London's *Daily Telegraph* on November 29, 2005. A fifteen-year-old girl living outside Quebec City had died after being admitted to the hospital for what was thought to be an anaphylactic reaction to peanuts. The reason? A passionate 3 a.m. kiss with her boyfriend—after he had eaten peanut butter. Her friends didn't even know of her allergy until they pulled an EpiPen from her backpack. She had a MedicAlert bracelet, but she did not wear it.

"If peanuts are still in the mouth, or on the tongue or on the lips, they can cause a reaction," said Dr. Karen Sigman, an allergy expert, in an interview for the *Telegraph*. "Teenagers with allergies have to let their friends know. If they are going to be dating somebody, then they have to tell the people they are close to that they are allergic to make sure they are not in contact with nuts or peanuts."

There was a precedent for suspicion that kissing had been the culprit. In 2003, the *Mayo Clinic Proceedings* had published a case report on a twenty-year-old woman who had been admitted to a hospital with lip angioedema (swelling), nausea, wheezing, cramps, and a significant drop in blood pressure, all of which had happened immediately after receiving a good-night kiss from her boyfriend. The girl had a known allergy to crustaceans; the boy had eaten shrimp less than an hour earlier. She had recovered, but only after receiving several treatments including prednisone, nebulized albuterol, and intravenous epinephrine.

"Kissing, an ancient technique for expressing simple affection or erotic desire, has been recognized only recently as a vector for transmitting food allergens," noted Dr. David P. Steensma, in his report. This was probably the only time Steensma has ever had to create a footnote citing William Cane's *The Art of Kissing*.

As Canadian coroner Michel Miron would announce in the spring of 2006, the case of the fifteen-year-old victim turned out to be a bit more complicated. The girl had a history of severe asthma as well as allergies, and had been spending hours at a party with smokers; there were traces of marijuana in her system. These factors had contributed to an asthma attack, rather than a food reaction, and the subsequent cerebral anoxia (when oxygen cannot reach your brain) that actually led to her death. Her boyfriend's snack of peanut butter and toast had been at 6 p.m., more than nine hours before they had kissed and she had begun complaining of shortness of breath.

"A study shows at the end of an hour, there is no allergen left in the saliva," Miron said at a press conference, paraphrasing the known science in order to spare the boy a lifetime of guilt.

That story touched off an international wave of interest in "kissing reactions." Mount Sinai School of Medicine staged an experiment in which volunteers ate two tablespoons of peanut butter in a sandwich. Subsequent interventions to neutralize the peanut allergens included brushing one's teeth, chewing gum, and rinsing the mouth out with water. While some subjects' mouths were clean of peanut proteins after nothing more than a five-minute wait (maybe people had not chewed thoroughly; maybe they harbored particularly aggressive saliva), some people had detectable traces of nut in their mouths more than three hours later. According to a study published in the *Journal of Allergy and Clinical Immunology*, the most foolproof way to avoid causing a reaction in a romantic partner—if you insist on eating something he or she is allergic to—is to wait four hours and chew on something "safe" before kissing.

Tell that to the guy picking you up for dinner and a movie on a Friday night.

A decade ago, as I entered my twenties, more and more friends began forwarding me articles on reactions caused by intimate contact, asking, "Have you heard of this?" Of course I had. I was the girl who, at my own ninth-grade Christmas party, had forced myself to veto a spin-the-bottle kiss from the guy I had a crush on. Why? Because he confessed he had eaten a handful of M&M's before the game had started.

Then there was the college boyfriend whose love affair with dairy had been entrenched long before I came onto the scene.

Once, during a particularly vicious fight at his house, he stalked out of the bedroom to cool off while I stayed in bed and fumed. He came back and we began making up—and making out. After a few minutes, I pulled away. Something was not right.

"Guess your allergies aren't *so* bad," he said.

He had used his time out of sight to snack on a square of chocolate. I ran to the bathroom and flipped on the light, to reveal that my collarbone was erupting in hives.

That relationship was not long for this world. But a guy doesn't have to be callous to cause harm; even simple carelessness poses a danger.

Before moving in together, Adam and I had spent a few years trying (and failing) to make a long-distance relationship work. He was still at the University of Virginia, attending law school, while I worked in D.C. as the assistant to a journalist. Both of us were strapped for cash and perpetually exhausted. On the weekends, we made long road trips to see each other, thinking it would keep the spark alive. Instead, we'd struggle to stay awake long enough to watch a rented movie on his laptop, which had a screen prone to reflective glare and a DVD drive that froze up every five minutes. Then we'd pass out on my too-small futon or the mattress he laid on the floor in lieu of a proper bed.

One Friday, having fought my way out of town despite a particularly grueling evening rush hour on Interstate 66, I marched into his house determined to have a "romantic" reunion. I ignored the trash bags piled by the front door. I ignored the fact that the living room reeked of citrus (courtesy of a construction-worker roommate who appeared to eat nothing but oranges, strewing piles of peel and pith around the house). I ignored the fact that Adam had just gotten back from the gym and was still in basketball shorts and sweaty T-shirt.

Ignoring it all, I hopped onto his lap, before he could get up from his hand-me-down plaid couch, and gave him a deep kiss.

I had also ignored my knowledge of Adam's habitual post-workout routine. After a second I tasted the chalky residue of milk on my tongue. I yanked back, pressing my palm to my lips, but it was too late. My mouth began to tingle.

"What did you have?" I asked, only then noticing the water glass filmed in white.

"Ovaltine," he said sheepishly.

"What are you, a grandmother?" I snapped.

I got off his lap and went to take a long drink of lukewarm water from the tap. The reaction could not be stopped. A Benadryl pill later, I settled in on the couch, lips apart so I could take in air even as my nasal passages shut down. Nothing more attractive than a pissed-off mouth-breather, I know.

"I'm sorry," he said. But I was madder at myself. So much for Date Night.

Every relationship revolves around issues of trust. We prioritize our individual expectations—in terms of religion, sex, family, money—and hope to find the person who can honor those needs. In every relationship there will be moments when that trust is broken. You can internalize your partner's reactions to these moments, picking and choosing when to flip out and when to let it go; most of the time I can, too. But I can't shrug off a lapse in judgment when it comes to handling my food allergies. Each violation is as undeniable as a hive on the cheek.

Those with allergies are forced into becoming custodians to the lifestyles of those around us. It's one thing to announce you're going on a diet and then sneak a cheeseburger on the side. That's your business. But when you then kiss me and I have to go to the hospital, even though you've allegedly been eating nothing but celery and hummus all week, your business becomes my problem.

So with Adam, and boyfriends before and since, I have to question ("Did you wash up?"). I have to quiz. I have to be meticulous about the other person's hygiene, at the risk of feeling less like a lover and more like a mom. And I can never get entirely swept up in the moment.

Cosmopolitan and *Glamour* hype the importance of good "chemistry" in a relationship. Not just conscious traits and habits but that ephemeral mix of hormones, pheromones, and every other kind of moan. Do my food allergies alter my chemistry? Should I be holding out for a neat freak? Looking for a vegan? Could I have stayed with Adam if he'd woken up one morning knowing his true calling was as a shrimp fisherman?

As if that wasn't enough to worry about, judging "chemistry" with a partner has an additional critical (if slightly vulgar) dimension. There's another kind of allergy people ask about. I'm going to demur on calling it a food allergy, but let me just say once and for all: Allergies are triggered by ingestion or exposure to proteins. Any proteins. Proteins found in food, pet dander, pollen.

Proteins found in sperm.

After you filter out all the misdiagnoses related to sexually transmitted diseases and chemical irritation, semen allergy is rare. But it exists. The first documented case was in 1958, when Dutch gynecologist J. L. H. Specken examined a sixty-five-year-old woman who experienced postcoital hives and bronchial spasms. The allergy is usually diagnosed among women in their twenties who have a known history of vaginitis unresponsive to other treatments. The marker for diagnosis is an absence of symptoms when condoms are used; a skin-prick test will confirm IgE-based response to seminal proteins.

This is one allergy I have never experienced firsthand. But that doesn't mean I think of it as the punch line to some dirty joke. Having struggled to be honest with a partner midkiss, I can't even fathom the stress of having to pull away in bed to say, "Um, I think we have a problem." The physical impact is as agonizing as any reaction. Not just burning and redness in any area of contact—which can last from hours to days—but wheezing and other systemic symptoms.

The long-term consequences are also intimidating. Once diagnosed with a semen allergy, a woman trying to conceive may have to begin taking prednisone in the seven to ten days prior to each predicted ovulation, to prime her body to handle the stress of unprotected sex. Anyone who has taken prednisone knows it is quite the mood killer, associated with rapid weight gain and extreme irritability. If that doesn't work, the couple may have to resort to the expense and complications of in vitro fertilization, even if they have otherwise healthy sperm and eggs.

There are a couple of desensitization treatments, preferably using materials taken from the likely sexual partner. One option is receiving shots containing small doses of the, er, allergen. The other method would be a "graded challenge," in which various dilutions of semen are placed in the vagina every twenty minutes, building up a tolerance to the whole and undiluted form.

Once tolerance is established, the allergy sufferer needs to maintain a certain minimum level of exposure to the allergen.

The recommendation: sexual intercourse no less than every forty-eight hours.

You could look at this as the silver lining. Unless you or your partner travels frequently, in which case medical necessity dictates the creation of some very unholy variations on the freezer pop, to be used in his absence.

. . .

My first date with Adam was in my second year of college. Not a date, really. More like a "Hey, Sandra, I'm grabbing a bite. Wanna come along?" Not exactly rose petals showered at my feet. But if you're a girl deep in the clutches of a crush, such an invitation trumps Prince Charming pulling up in his gilded carriage.

We had gone to Café Europa, a popular hangout on the Corner known for cheap Mediterranean sandwiches served deli-style from behind a glass counter. Souvlaki, falafel, feta, and eggplant: the messy, greasy comfort foods that help a nineteen-year-old power through a ten-page sociology paper or a raging hangover. The café's logo, a woman with a strong nose and wiggly lines for hair—presumably Europa—looked like it had been doodled with a Bic pen on someone's napkin. The plates were paper, the forks plastic.

"Can you find something here?" Adam had asked.

"Sure!" I'd said brightly. "I love this place."

Actually, I'd never eaten there. Its student staff, while friendly, didn't seem overly diligent about avoiding cross-contamination or contamination, period. I waited for Adam to get his order and then sent him off to grab a table while I asked question after question of the guy behind the counter.

I settled on hummus, carrot and celery sticks, and wedges of pita, setting my plate down on a table that wobbled to the touch. The hummus was a bad move—grainy, garlicky, an eminently unfit premise to a kiss. But I soon had much bigger problems.

Bubbles. I tried to ignore the sensation of pockets of air rising from behind my sternum, working their way painfully up my windpipe, popping, rising again. Focusing on eye contact with Adam, I took a long sip of a Coke that had been mixed with too much sweet cola syrup. Pop. Pop. Pop.

This had to be a minor reaction, a contamination issue as predicted. Carrots and chickpeas were harmless. The manager had sworn up and down that the pita contained no dairy. (Later, I'd find out the staff did not consider goat's milk a form of "dairy.")

Adam was making small talk about movies. It was all I could do to stay upright, nod, smile, swallow, smile again. Occasionally I would trace my fingertips over my cheeks, hoping it looked like a flirtatious gesture as I felt for radiant heat or hives. *At least,* I thought, *my skin isn't getting all blotchy. Yet.*

Forty minutes passed in a blur. We walked back together to Alderman Library, where he was meeting a study group. Only after I saw the doors close behind him did I walk to the building next door, find a pay phone, and call the University Hospital. I was in an ambulance soon after.

I've always been quick to hide a reaction if I can get away with it. Sometimes it's because I'm embarrassed by the cause.

One evening, at the age of ten, I was feeding my kitten bits of dried cat food—flicking it across the laundry room floor so he would chase after it—and without even thinking, put a piece on my tongue. Dried milk, beef extract, shrimp protein, who knows what else: gulp. Gone. I *squonked* my way through dinner that night, while insisting to my mother that everything was fine.

Even under more dignified circumstances, there is an element of pride. I want to be with someone who cares about me, not someone who considers himself a caretaker. As far as dates go, allergy attacks aren't pretty. A reaction is no dainty "spell" that leaves me dabbing at my mouth with a handkerchief. There will be gasping and sweating and retching. Getting ready to go out for a dinner date, I always line and shadow my eyelids knowing that by the end of the night they could be swollen and heavy with fluid. I coat my lips in Chapstick, not knowing if I'll end up with a kiss or mouth-to-mouth from a fifty-three-year-old paramedic with halitosis.

Eight years and several breakups after that ill-fated Café Europa meal, Adam and I would once again be sitting down to eat together—this time in D.C., in a diner called Open City, across the street from an apartment he'd rented in my neighborhood. By then, I'd gone on enough dates to know to steer clear of bread entirely. Still, a few bites into my salad, I felt that familiar tickle.

I got up to use the restroom, taking a long look back into the kitchen as I passed. I could see that while the men were wearing gloves as they mixed the greens, they were not changing gloves between salads. Which meant that the residual oil from someone's handful of cheddar was now all over the roasted red peppers on my plate.

Returning to the table, I nibbled on another leaf or two, then pretended I was full. As Adam walked me back to my place, my mask of composure slipped. I slowed, then staggered. I leaned against a metal railing, sure I would throw up on the street.

"Let's get home," I said. "I need to get home."

Once in the door, I ran to the bathroom, hunching down as my guts roiled. Adam waited outside. Every few minutes he would call in, "Are you okay?"

I was determined to be okay. I couldn't let Adam see this, but I couldn't let him leave me alone, either. The second Benadryl was failing to take hold. I felt dizzy.

"Are you okay?"

I heard the question, but couldn't shape a response. As sometimes happens with bad reactions, a surreal image was rising up in my head. This time it was my breath as the bow on a violin, being drawn back and forth. Back . . . forth . . . back . . .

Keep playing, I thought hazily. *Play.*

That was when the bathroom door nearly jumped off its hinges as he busted in.

"GET OUT," I hollered, trying to yank up my underwear.

Relieved that I was conscious, Adam quickly stepped back into the hallway and closed the door.

Later, after the EMT team had come and gone, he sat down next to me on the spindly futon I was still calling my bed. He wrapped his arms around me.

"Do me a favor," he said. "Don't die."

My posture stayed stiff, resisting his hug. I was mortified at the view he'd gotten in the bathroom.

"Sandra," he said. "You have to understand. I couldn't picture explaining to your mom that I let you die alone—and on a toilet."

That was when I knew he intended to stick around for a while. Yet even after we'd known each other so long that we were ready to try sharing a household, I don't think he was prepared for the thousand minor hassles of living with my food allergies. Not just the allergies themselves but a personality shaped by a lifetime of managing those allergies.

I am a compulsive double-checker and to-do lister, a scrutinizer of labels and a labeler of file folders. In contrast, Adam followed the philosophy of open-air filing, in which anything is easier to find if you leave it in plain view. This goes for bills, socks, used water glasses, and month-old crossword puzzles. He moved through the apartment like a poltergeist, leaving every conceivable cabinet and drawer hanging ajar in his wake.

It's not as if I didn't have some warning. Throughout college, he would snack on a jar of peanut butter that he kept in his room, open, with a knife stuck into it for handy serving. Each time I visited, the jar had roamed to a different spot—the bedside stand, the dresser, the seat of a chair. I called it his free-range peanut butter.

Even as a grown-up, he was still a grown-up *guy*. He harbored half-empty soda cans, scooped with the same spoon from the Nutella to the ice cream and back again, and kept three tubs of cottage cheese in simultaneous rotation. When it was his kitchen, at his place, I could ignore a sticky counter or a dirty dish. But once his kitchen became mine, it wasn't just a matter of habits that made my skin crawl. These were habits that could make my skin break out into hives, or worse.

"Did you get all the eggs off that plate?" I'd say. "You kind of have to scrub before you load it in the dishwasher, or else they get baked on."

"Um, can you throw that milk away? That's still in the fridge? I'm pretty sure it has gone over," I'd point out. "You know I can't touch it."

For the one being nagged, it had to have been awful. My allergies leverage every concern—both legitimate grievances and, I confess, occasional mere PMS bitchery—into a litmus test. *Do you love me? Then rinse out that glass.*

Sometimes I wonder if I'm destined to live alone. Otherwise, I'll have to accept this reality in which once or twice every week I break out in hives in my own house. It might happen when I swipe away a drop of orange juice, only to realize the counter is also coated in a fine drift of whey powder from my significant other's protein shakes. It might be when I surprise him with a kiss, only to hear too late, "I had cream in my coffee."

Then again, I'm not the only one making a compromise in such a household. Any partner has to accept a reality in which there will be many nights when I am curled up, gasping and heaving, on the other side of a door. Nights in which it flashes through his head, *What will I say to her mother if she dies?*

Just a few months after Adam and I had moved in together, I went out by myself for a friend's "salon" dinner—a gathering of people from D.C.'s literary world, all friends of hers, all strangers to one another. When I came to the door, she handed me a cheat sheet that had every guest's name typed out in curly pink script. At first the guests tried to match faces to names and names to jobs as we stood around in her cute Georgetown living room. We soon abandoned the obligatory networking and moved on to admiring her poodle, a regal descendant of a Westminster prizewinner.

Our hostess set down a plate of warm pastry puffs. The dog sniffed them delicately before turning away. I reached out to try a puff, thinking I recognized the type as one I bought regularly at Trader Joe's. Then realized these were filled with shrimp. Close call. My stomach growled.

When dinner was served, I walked over and grabbed a plate. I got the rundown on how the pork loin had been prepared. Olive oil, herbs, heat; it seemed perfect. But seconds after swallowing the first bite of mango-topped pork, my throat began to itch.

Oh no. This was back when I still thought mango was safe. I'd had juice blended with mango and had tested out mango salsa without a hitch. But after those first two exposures, apparently my system had changed its mind. My gut cramped. I unzipped my purse, slivered the foil of a Benadryl with my thumbnail, and palmed the pill into my mouth. Looking around, I realized no one had noticed. Perhaps I could keep it that way.

I took another sip of wine, testing my ability to swallow. The hostess's poodle seemed to sense something was wrong. She settled in at my side and nosed my hand. I'd fallen silent for too long.

Taking a deep breath and turning to the playwright on my left, I asked, "So, when did you leave England?"

He answered with a long story, but it was hard to focus. The throat itch wasn't going away. Maybe I could coat my stomach with something bland, but there was no helpful bowl of pretzels handy. This was too fancy a party for that. The French bread, handmade, was also of indeterminate ingredients. Broiled salmon?

I got up and served myself two filets, then part of a third, eating it with my fingers from a plate still full of mango and pork. I looked like a total glutton, but it worked. The itch eased.

"So you live with your boyfriend?" the hostess asked.

"Yes," I told them, "Adam. He's a lawyer." I talked about meeting him in college, leaving out that our first date ended with me alone in the ER. I was determined to make it through the night without being labeled the Allergy Girl.

When it was time for dessert, I oohed and aahed with everyone else at the dozen assorted cupcakes, though I couldn't actually imagine how they would taste. The thin bakery box began making its way around the table, and I noticed the cardboard bottom was seeped through with butter frosting. I faked digging something out of my purse as it passed, to avoid touching it.

The guests walked out together. I was so grateful to have held the reaction at bay that I didn't even flinch when the journalist's wife gave me a frostinged kiss good night. I settled behind the wheel, feeling the kiss-shaped hive begin to rise on my cheek.

I walked in to find Adam on the floor, playing Star Wars on his Xbox. I leaned down for a kiss hello and he gestured to the open jar of Nutella.

"I'm deadly," he warned. "How was dinner?"

"It was fun," I told him, "until the reaction." There was no need to pretend anymore. The Benadryl was wearing off. I could feel a return of tickling in my throat.

"That sucks." If I was well enough to talk, Adam had learned not to press for details. He looked back at the screen. "Want to watch me kill some droids?"

"Sure," I said. "If I throw up, it's not editorial." I took another Benadryl, knowing it would knock me out, and curled up in the recliner.

They don't show this in the Hollywood romances: how the whooshing of lightsabers can become a lullaby. How you hope your true love will be someone you trust to check on your breathing as you sleep.

. . .

In high school, I had my first hint that weddings might prove hazardous to my health. The object of my affection, a Hindu, joked one day about the Bengali tradition of the Bou Bhat ceremony. Upon arrival at the groom's house, he told me, women wash the bride's feet in flour and milk.

"Milk?" I asked, sure I had misheard.

Yep. Alternately, the bride could simply step into the mixture, imprinting her soles, before being led into the house—where she would be fed sherbet. Or, as I like to think of sherbet, "sweet icy death in a bowl."

I went home that night and did some research. As in all cultures where food is prized, the *sanskara* of Indian weddings features allergen after allergen. The *madhupak*, in which the father of the bride was supposed to offer the groom yogurt and honey in welcome. The casting of ghee, clarified butter, into the fire we would circle four times.

None of this would come to pass. My allergy to these rites

was just the literal manifestation of a larger incongruity. His parents would never have approved of their son marrying "that white girl."

Still I was intrigued. I'd never thought about weddings before. I began cataloguing a variety of matrimonial cultural traditions, filing each under *fun* or *fatal*. In Morocco, the bride's body is bathed in milk (to purify her) before applying henna to her hands and feet. In Italy and Greece, the couple is showered with sugared almonds as they walk to the limousine. In the Czechoslovakian tradition, they were showered with peas instead. In Hungary, the bride smashes an egg to ensure the health of her future children. In Bulgaria, the bride puts an egg in a dish with wheat and coins and tosses it over her head.

All of these scenarios were, for me, strictly hypothetical. Then, after college graduation, I had the first of my Summer of a Thousand Weddings: those seasons when it seems like every weekend involves putting on a semiformal dress, making small talk with someone's uncle, and dancing to the Isley Brother's "Shout" after too many glasses of champagne. At this point in my life I realized I had a very real, very tangible foe when it came to the battlefield of matrimony. Enemy, thy name is cake.

The tradition of wedding cakes supposedly goes back to ancient Rome, when the groom broke a "cake" (that is, a loaf) of barley bread over the bride's head as evidence of her submission. A gentler version describes him crumbling it over her to suggest fertility. I suspect the reality could go either way depending on a couple's dynamic, just as the sharing of first bites today can consist of loving forkfuls or a mutual face-smush.

By the middle of the seventeenth century, and with sugar still unavailable to many, the cake had evolved into a "bride's pye" used in European wedding ceremonies. The Chinese took to serving dragon and phoenix cakes, individually portioned and usually filled with red or green adzuki-bean paste—a tradition that continues today. Some bride's-pie recipes ordained ingredients that doubled as aphrodisiacs, including oysters, cockscombs, and lamb testicles. Thankfully, cooks dumped in enough spice to cover the actual flavor. Simpler versions used mincemeat or fruit and nuts.

Sometimes a glass ring would be embedded inside the cake. Whoever found it would be blessed with good luck in the coming year. Unless you found it by swallowing it, in which case the luck was suspect.

Today, different cake traditions abound. The French *croque-en-bouche* is textured in chocolate-dipped profiteroles stuffed with pastry cream, or ganache-filled macarons; picture a pastry-covered wizard's hat, threaded in caramel. The Norwegian *kransekake* also takes on a conical appearance, as marzipan rings of gradually decreasing size are stacked, one on top of the other, sometimes around a bottle of wine. In Appalachia, people serve "stack cake," a series of thin layers contributed by each of the attending guest parties, iced together with a swipe of apple butter or preserves. Stack cakes (named so because they end up looking like a stack of pancakes) double as a social barometer. The more popular the couple, the taller their cake.

These variations, plus the tiered classics of vanilla sponge cake, chocolate sponge cake, or carrot cake, all have one thing in common: they would kill me.

While passing on having a slice is easy enough, it doesn't eliminate the threat. At every wedding I find myself surrounded by dozens of people, intoxicated to varying degrees, whose fingers and lips are now coated with something that will bring tears to my eyes and hives to my cheeks. I become Frogger, trying to cross from our table to the door without being hit by the Mack trucks of every handshake, hug, and kiss.

I approach every wedding prepared for battle. I pack extra Benadryl. I check the expiration date on my EpiPen. I say "No thanks," over and over, to trays held out by smiling waiters. I sneak peanut butter pretzels during the appetizers. I have two men who, because we share the same crowd of old high-school friends, are frequently invited to the same weddings. They are my stunt eaters, always willing to take a few bites of my surf or turf so that my plate does not go completely untouched. Even with those precautions in place, out of the twenty-plus ceremonies I have attended, more than a dozen have culminated in an allergic reaction.

At one wedding, I took a gamble on nibbling at a slice of tomato and two pieces of lettuce that had been served to me as a "special plate." The same knife that had sliced my tomato had probably been used on the mozzarella served in everyone else's *insalata caprese*. The band began to play, and a literature professor from my graduate program invited me to dance. We made it through one round of swing steps and slow turns.

Then I had my Cinderella moment—running from the ballroom, shawl trailing on the ground behind me, and finding the guest restroom in the hotel just in time. I'd knelt down to the toilet, ignoring the scrunch of my satin dress against the tile, and heaved.

For the next hour I would sit in the fancy lobby, a rotation of friends and classmates keeping me company as I waited for my breath to stabilize for the walk home. Strains of big-band music could still be heard through the doors to the reception.

"Maybe I'm just allergic to weddings," I said to one girl.

Then one of my best friends from college became engaged to a vegetarian. Stephanie was bound and determined that I not just have a complete meal after their ceremony, but that I have dessert. She sent me an email with a list of cake batter ingredients that ranged from the commonplace (salt and vanilla) to the quirky (oat flour and Florida Crystals Evaporated Cane Juice). When it became clear that the only deal breaker in her wedding cake was the frosting's soy, she negotiated with the baker, asking if they could do an unfrosted cupcake on the side. The baker one-upped by offering to make a dairy-free, soy-free ganache with vegan dark chocolate.

"Can you have any of those things?" Steph wrote to me. "Or would it be too scary to have this stuff?"

I thought about admitting that, yes, it was too scary. Did I even have a taste for chocolate? But she seemed so excited, and she had gone to all that trouble.

"Let's give it a shot," I wrote back.

On the big day, the bride found me minutes after the cake cutting. This was usually right around the time I start edging toward the exit. At first I assumed she was coming to apologize, empty-handed, but instead (as if she'd had it hidden in the folds of her wedding gown), with a flourish Steph materialized my very own cupcake, swirled in dark-brown frosting.

I waited until she'd left to take a tiny bite, sure that something would go wrong. But my *Hmmm* turned into an *Mmmm*.

The cake's interior was sweet, moist, and 100 percent Sandra-friendly. Good lord.

The next morning, I called my mother. Skipping over the weather, the guests, how beautiful Steph had looked, blahblahblah—I cut to the chase. "I have to tell you about this cupcake," I said.

"It worries me," my mother admitted the other day, thinking of the wedding she'd like for me to be able to have. I don't have a fiancé lined up, but my mother is already clipping articles on vegan bakeries that might be able to replicate Steph's cupcake. She brainstorms substitutes for mini-quiches and deviled eggs. "After all," she says, "it's not like someone with your allergies can just send out pigs in a blanket."

This is not a woman who has ever romanticized being the mother of the bride. She married my father in the chapel of Vinson Hall, a retirement community close to her parents' home in McLean, Virginia. Afterward, they served punch and cookies in the community's recreation room, right next to the pool tables. This was after her sister's wedding, which was held in the family garage, papered over and painted to look like a garden. When *their* mother had gotten married, the thing my grandmother always talked about was not the hors d'oeuvres, or the dress, but rather the months it took beforehand for Carl, my grandfather, to save up the gas to drive them to their honeymoon.

I ask my mother what kind of cake she had at Vinson Hall.

"Yellow sheet . . . something," she says. "What I really remember is being starved and never getting the chance to eat anything."

With no inherited wedding-diva streak, it's hard to come to terms with the fact that unless I want the official wedding portrait to show the bride on a stretcher, the day really will have to revolve around my needs. I will have to choose a venue that is not handling any other catered events that day, to avoid the risk of cross-contamination in the kitchen. I will have to find the caterer who doesn't blink when I ask them to list every single cooking oil they will use. I will need to see every recipe, every label. I will hunt down either my friend's baker or another one who knows how to make the base of ganache with coconut milk. The guy can have his choice of groom's cake—but only to the extent of selecting from groom's cakes that also happen to be Sandra-friendly. Maybe we won't even serve cream with the coffee.

I'm probably setting myself up for a high-stakes disaster. I should trade it in for a city hall ceremony and some really amazing sushi afterward. Yet part of me dreams of having an evening when all my loved ones eat the way I eat every day—and everyone eats well, and everyone leaves full, and there's not one moment of pity.

Just once, I want to fight someone for that last bite of cake.

CHAPTER EIGHT

On the Road

When my sister first moved off campus during her college years, she found a group apartment in New York
City's East Village, down the street from the KGB Bar. Her
apartment was perfumed in the distilled essence of cigarettes
and had Christmas lights strung up year-round, couches upholstered in stained 1920s velvet, and jug bottles of merlot. Someone had transformed the chandelier into an installation piece,
complete with birds' nests and a steady swarm of gnats.

It was the perfect space for artistic Manhattanites who—
used to the pendulum swing between windfall gigs and
unemployment—could champion two-hundred-dollar shoes
and bedside stands salvaged from the curb with equal enthusiasm. One morning, my sister opened her bedroom door to find
a three-model *Playboy* shoot being staged in the living room.

Most mornings, she opened the door to a dog urine puddle between the living room couch and the sideboard she used as a dresser.

On a visit to New York, I went with Christina and her boyfriend to her favorite neighborhood restaurant for dinner before catching the 9 p.m. train back to D.C. The Asian-deco bistro offered design-your-own rice bowls and seven-dollar *aguas frescas*. Like many places in the Village, it favored vegetarians, meaning that it wasn't easy to avoid soy. When my throat protested after the third or fourth bite of my rice bowl, I figured it was the whole edamame I'd tried to pick around in the veggie slaw, or maybe soy mayo providing the creamy base to garlic-ginger "sauce." I switched my attention to the rainbow of rice to choose from—coconut, Bhutanese red, Forbidden black—and took a long swig of my ginger-laced juice. The reaction subsided.

If I'd known that shrimp had been listed among the half dozen ingredients of the dumplings we'd shared as an appetizer (as Christina's boyfriend later remembered it), I might have been more alarmed. Or I might have shrugged it off. I'd had only one dumpling, and as far as I knew, it was not a potent allergy. As a child I'd enjoyed shrimp tempura. Only a few nights of suspicious mouth-tingling responses, beginning around the age of twelve, plus a natural wariness of shellfish, had led me to deem shrimp off-limits.

After dinner I cabbed it to Penn Station, grabbed a window seat on the Northeast Regional, and was asleep within minutes. Around 11 p.m. I jolted awake, my eyes struggling to open despite sore and gluey contact lenses. Where was I? My throat hurt.

I was in the grip of a biphasic reaction, my mast cells

responding with renewed vigor hours after the initial allergen exposure. These reactions are an unwelcome novelty that began occurring in my late twenties. They are triggered by cashews, mango, and (as I was now learning) shrimp. There was a possibility of vomiting, diarrhea, even anaphylaxis. And I was stuck on an Amtrak train, with an hour between me and D.C.

I got my phone out and dialed home, hoping to connect with Adam to see if he could meet me at the train station. No answer. I was too jittery to compose a sensible text message. I dialed again. When it went to voice mail, the words poured out.

"Adam it's me and I'm having a really bad reaction and if you can—"

In my hunched-over position, sprawled across two seats, a uniformed waist filled my field of vision. I looked up to find the conductor leaning down intently.

"Excuse me, miss."

I kept talking into the phone. "... someone just came up, maybe ..." I thought he'd seen my distress and was asking if I needed a doctor's assistance.

"Miss."

"Yes." Maybe they would stop the train?

"Hang up that phone." Huh?

"Hang up *right now*. You are in the Quiet Car."

I snapped my phone shut. "Sir, I'm in the middle of a medical emergency. An allergic reaction."

He narrowed his eyes. "To what?"

"To ... my dinner," I said, knowing it sounded like a lie. Hours earlier, when I handed him my ticket, I'd seemed fine. I *had* been fine. He shook his head.

"Miss, I'm not going to ask you again. If you need to call

someone, then you step out of my car. I'll be watching you." He continued down the aisle, as a passenger two rows away gave me a cool stare over the top of his newspaper. Everyone in the seats around me had heard our conversation. No one asked if I needed help.

Sorry. Will call, I texted Adam. It would be another ten minutes before I felt up to walking to the next car. For now I got out my inhaler, shook it, puffed, shook it, puffed again—one part necessity, one part a desire to prove I wasn't faking. I dry swallowed a Benadryl. Then I doubled over in the seat and pressed my fists against my eyes. If there is an upside to tears, it's that they return moisture to dried-out contacts.

After years of being on the road with food allergies, I've come to expect exchanges with personnel who are at best puzzled, at worst surly. Case in point: for years, my mother would send me off on any trip longer than two days with a whole loaf of Giant-brand Italian bread in my suitcase, as insurance that I would never risk eating something contaminated because I had no other option.

Try explaining that to the airport security guard who found an eight-inch serrated knife in my bag as my high school choir waited to board our flight for Disney World. You know, for cutting the bread. She held it up in the air, calling out for its owner. Even now I can picture my mother's careful packing, folding a paper towel eight times over to serve as a sheath for the blade, securing it at top and bottom with a rubber band. Toothbrush, pajamas, underwear, big knife; wasn't this how everyone packed?

On vacations, my family would pay extra for a fridge and microwave, and travel by car whenever possible. My father was always the one behind the wheel. My mother liked to fill an entire suitcase with Sandra-friendly food, right down to her own dish detergent, sponges, salt and pepper shakers, and a small water bottle filled with cooking oil. (They would also tuck in a small water bottle filled with vodka, but I didn't figure this out until years later.)

When packing our food was not possible, she'd insist that a grocery store be our first stop, sometimes even before we had checked into our hotel. My father would keep the rental car running in the parking lot, rolling the window down so he could drum his fingers impatiently on the door. She'd come back with "just the essentials," e.g., orange juice, a box of Corn Pops, peanut butter, pretzels, frozen peas or lima beans, a pack of bacon, dried linguine, a roll of paper towels, a box of Kleenex, and a tin of cashews or macadamias. I couldn't eat the nuts. They were for my father—a peace offering.

For years, my dad, in his civilian life as a lawyer, has counseled a Hawaiian nonprofit that protects the interests of native Pacific islanders. This meant periodic weeks of meetings in Oahu; for several years, we joined him, traveling to additional islands and turning the business trip into a family vacation. With each visit we became more at home. We no longer needed to cut the intensity of Kona coffee with decaf. We had been through all fourteen climates of the Big Island. We took to returning to a favorite rental complex in Maui, a Lahaina cove where turtles lived and bananas grew by the manager's office. By the time I was in my midtwenties, one of the few major Hawaii to-dos that remained undone, in our book, was Maui's Road to Hana.

The Road to Hana is a sixty-eight-mile stretch of Hawaiian

state highway known for its tropical rain forest and its sharp curves, more than six hundred of them, which connects the populous center of Kahului with the tiny town of Hana. The trip crosses fifty-nine bridges, most of which are century-old concrete, at least forty-six of which are one lane. Two cars meeting head-on have to spontaneously determine who has right of way—or else play chicken.

The trip was rumored to be both epic and exhausting. Most tourists, upon arrival in Hana, start planning their return trip within hours. Otherwise they risk getting stranded by darkness. The locals call them "whizzers."

If the possibility of taking the Road to Hana had been raised on earlier trips, my mother must have vetoed it. She believes men (e.g., my father) are innately programmed to find a beautiful beach spot, rent a house . . . and then plan day after day of activities that prevent anyone (e.g., my mother) from getting to lie out in the sun, relax, and read even one of the three paperback novels she would have optimistically packed in her luggage. Car trips were a necessary evil, not an adventure. *Besides,* I could imagine her saying to my dad, *who knows where we'll find a restaurant for Sandra?*

But on this particular trip, the scales had tipped. I was older, confident in my ability to navigate any café menu. My mother managed to sunburn her chest on the first day, making the lounge chair less appealing. My father had invited along his law partner, James, who had brought his girlfriend Kim, and they had rented a black convertible whose suspension was tailor-made for six hundred–plus tight turns. My father had made sure our rental could keep up, upgrading to a six-cylinder engine. We were going.

We'd been warned it was a three-hour drive. It seemed impossible that sixty-some miles could take that long. Yet after the first hour, it was clear we had no control over our speed, since there were no passing lanes—and no option of turning back, since there were no intersections. The rusted vans and pickups ahead of us seemed to be running on molasses. The only thing worse were the cars driven by the island's resident meth-head population, periodically barreling down on us in the opposite direction.

After one near sideswipe by a powder-blue lowrider (the driver wild-eyed and flashing us his middle finger, his seven-year-old son grinning from the passenger seat), we saw a hand-made sign for TWIN FALLS. We pulled over, grateful for the chance to stretch our legs.

"How far to the water?" we asked a family threading their way out of the woods.

"Not too far," they said.

The trek turned out to be a half mile (balancing single-file on an iron train tie at one point), culminating in the chance to jump into the falls or swing out, by rope, over a natural pool. It was beautiful, but it made clear how isolated we were from the accoutrements of tourism. We'd expected signage for other scenic spots—the tide pools, the black-sand beaches—but this hand-scrawled piece of cardboard was as close as we'd get. There were no restrooms, no stands where I could buy fresh pineapple for a snack, and no places to get film or bug spray.

Back in the car, we were lulled into silence by the increasingly exotic foliage revealed with each switchback. For a long stretch, the Road to Hana threads along a canyon drop-off straight out of the Jurassic era. We passed through a patch of "painted" rainbow gum trees, each trunk's pedestrian-gray outer bark peeling off to reveal patches of mint green, neon pink, and orange.

On the road went . . . and went . . . and went. I slouched down so my sister could tip her head against my shoulder, and she dozed off. Sometimes we'd zip over a bridge, not realizing until we'd crossed it that we had missed a place to pull over and see a waterfall.

"We'll stop on the way back," my mother said hopefully.

We were ready for Hana. We were now snaking along open coast, hundreds of feet above sea level, with the occasional small village twinkling far below. We hadn't passed a single restaurant. I had eaten as many almonds as I could manage and had drunk two cans of soda, and my stomach was still growling.

A few minutes into Hour Four, we passed the first sign we'd seen in ten miles.

THE ROAD TO HANA IS ABOUT THE JOURNEY, NOT THE DESTINATION, it said.

This was a nice way of warning that when you arrive in Hana, what you'll find is a dowdy stretch of dirt road. The "Historic Courthouse and Jail" turned out to be a wooden shack with an outhouse that was designed to be padlocked from the outside. Did it double as a jail cell?

A deep-tanned man in a torn T-shirt sat in a pickup truck in the otherwise deserted parking lot. We asked where we could get a meal.

"There's one place," he said, pointing down the road. "Hana Ranch."

We piled back in the car. But before we could make the prescribed turn, my father spotted what seemed to be a gas station, the first in hours. Not sure how late it would stay open, he overruled our objections and steered toward it.

Rounding a hill, a huge lava-rock cross loomed to our right: Fagan's Cross, a memorial to the man who brought cattle ranching to Hana.

"Oh my God," I said. "It's gorgeous."

I wasn't talking about the cross. To our left, just beyond the station, was a collection of creamy-walled, thatch-roofed buildings, a curving private driveway, and an ornate, multitier fountain. We had stumbled across the Hotel Hana-Maui and Honua Spa, which has to be the most incongruously located four-star resort in the United States.

Another time we might have hesitated to walk in, given our wrinkled clothes and our dusty shoes, but we were too grateful to be self-conscious, and they were too deserted to be snooty. There was a gift shop. There was a marble-floored ladies' room. Everywhere there were big, fresh flower arrangements of protea and birds-of-paradise. Within minutes we were seated in the Paniolo Lounge's big, soft chairs, menus in our laps.

"Will you be having drinks this evening?" the waiter asked.

"Yes," chorused every adult in unison.

If only the story ended after they brought that round of drinks to the table, complete with an umbrella for Christina's lemonade. Or if the story ended with the food, including the salad I'd ordered (determined to stay on my bikini diet), and the Kobe burgers that had James and my father raving over their flavor. Or even with the French fries I'd given in and ordered on the side, upon resolving that no one should try to diet on a road trip.

Unfortunately, after I ate my fries, I ate my mother's. After I ate hers, James held his plate out toward me.

"You want these?" he asked.

I took them. Was I even hungry at that point? Or was I just on Allergy Girl autopilot, eating for the ride home? I took them from his burger-tainted plate, and I ate them.

Ten minutes later, it was Christina who pointed out that I'd grown quiet, breathing shallowly and quickly through my mouth. They moved me from the plushy chair in the restaurant to a plushy chair in the lobby; I remember the firm press of upholstery against my back, and not much else. The concierge brought me cup after cup of cold water, poured from a pitcher garnished with hibiscus.

My father spoke in hushed tones with the hotel manager, who confirmed his fear. If things got worse, there was no emergency medical facility in Hana. To the east, there was only Charles Lindbergh's grave and miles of deserted national park.

We would have to leave right away, and we would have to take the road back the way we came.

My father is a decorated army veteran. There are plenty of stories out there to prove his stoicism under fire. But there has to be a special medal for making a three-hour drive in the dark, his oldest daughter in the backseat in a Benadryled haze—and not one hairpin turn he can afford to miss.

. . .

If traveling with food allergies within the country is difficult, traveling outside the country can be harrowing. Not to mention expensive, if something goes wrong. Most health insurance does not cover travel outside the United States, and most add-on international insurance plans do not cover allergic reactions, because they are considered a preexisting condition—even if they have never been previously diagnosed. Using your first time in Tokyo to try sea urchin? Probably not the best idea, if you have any history of seafood allergies. Neither is sampling the street food in Bangkok, no matter how mind-blowing Anthony Bourdain proclaims it to be.

The simplest dictate is that you should not venture into an area where your allergen is pervasive in the cuisine. I will never go to southern India, where everything from the roti to the tandoori chicken is made with dairy. But in northern India, where coconut milk is used instead, I could probably fare well.

In December 2001, our family's upcoming trip to Italy got a lot less scary once my father spoke to a native who assured him that flurrying every dish in Parmesan is an Italian-American affectation, and not the way of the old country. In fact, Italian tradition specifically prohibits serving fish and cheese together. (There is no definitive reason behind the taboo; if asked, many chefs state that it is because the pungency of cheese will overwhelm the delicate flavor of fish. My favorite theory is that because Italy's premiere cheese-making regions—Piedmont, Lombardy, Emilia-Romagna—are landlocked, the two specialties never met until many of Italy's culinary traditions had already been set.)

I've outgrown packing loaves of bread and eight-inch knives when I travel. Instead, I arm myself with a slip of paper, worded in whatever the common language is of the land I am visiting, that outlines my allergy issues. There are companies that will create these for you, such as Allerglobal and SelectWisely, usually for eight to nine dollars a pop. I'd skip that. The more generic and commercialized the warning appears, the less closely (I think) the waiter reads it. Besides, you don't want to bring a laminated card you have to fuss over retrieving. You want to bring a disposable, dispensable stack. They are business cards, in the sense that you are in the business of surviving this meal.

You can use one of those free online translation programs to create the text, but make sure to get it proofed by someone who speaks the language. There's a world of difference between handing someone a slip of paper that explains "Eggs are bad for me," and handing them a note that declares "My eggs are bad." It's helpful, too, to offer a few constructive guidelines; e.g., a list of oils that can be used to cook your food safely.

Even when there is not a language barrier, there are cultural obstacles to discerning reactions. In the United States, if someone were to begin wheezing and clutching at his throat soon after eating fish, eggs, or cow's milk, bystanders might leap to the possibility of allergic reaction and respond appropriately. They will know to call an ambulance and check the victim's bag for Benadryl or an epinephrine injector. Our awareness is primed. But the British, whose allergies to these foods are relatively uncommon, might not make the same logical leap. On the other hand, discomfort after eating hazelnuts—or peaches or apples—would raise the red flag.

Back to Italy. When my cousin Sara became engaged to Roderico, a member of the Arma dei Carabinieri, we were determined to attend their New Year's Eve 2001 wedding in Rome. Sara helped my mother translate a paragraph that listed my allergies. We rented a cold-water flat that included a full kitchen. I invited my then boyfriend to make the trip with us. I was a romantic, excited at the thought of having a real date to the black-tie ceremony at the Hotel Majestic Roma (the same hotel that, forty years earlier, had provided background scenes for Fellini's *La Dolce Vita*). My boyfriend, a Francophile, was excited at being there on the day Italy changed over to the euro.

Upon arriving in Rome, we picked up the rental car, a European model that fit all five of us only after some elaborate clown contortions. We got on the road and promptly almost missed our first two roundabout exits. It was then my father admitted, begrudgingly, that his eyesight was "a little off." He had gotten laser eye surgery less than two weeks before—without telling any of us—meaning he could only barely make out the signs in English, much less Italian. My boyfriend was unexpectedly drafted to play navigator to the very grumpy Brigadier General Beasley.

The evening of the wedding, I put on a long, black velvet column dress. We all crammed into the car once more, finding our way to Via Vittorio Veneto and the Majestic. It was easy to imagine Anita Ekberg skipping down the marble steps that anchored the hotel's Palladian facade. Inside, the salmon-pink walls of the room where Sara and Rodie were to be married shimmered with gold stenciling and sage-green draperies. Almost all of the family on my mother's side had made the flight overseas. We toasted a successful trip. Sara and Rodie said "I do." We drank more wine.

The wedding dinner was an elaborate, multicourse feast. Sara had worked painstakingly with the caterers to ensure a special meal for me, and everything was perfect up until the dessert—a cup of fresh fruit that someone, without even thinking, had strewn with butter-toasted almonds. I took two bites, then a Benadryl, before excusing myself to the bathroom. It was another fifteen minutes, when I had not returned, before my boyfriend figured out something was wrong.

I don't think I actually went to the bathroom. All I remember is taking another Benadryl and creeping off into one of the hotel's side parlors, where I sat down on a tufted satin couch. I deliberated with great intensity over whether the potted dwarf mandarin-orange tree beside the couch was real. I tore off a couple of leaves to check, rolling them between my fingers, sniffing. Then I curled up and passed out.

I woke up to find my mother sitting next to me on the couch, her fingers cupped over my warm forehead. My arm was asleep from serving as a pillow for my head. I'd drawn my knees up within my dress, stretching the velvet out of shape.

"Did you tell anyone?" I asked. "Don't tell anyone."

My father came over and crouched down, his dress uniform hunching up awkwardly around his shoulders.

"Do you need me to take you in?" he asked. "It's absolutely no problem if you want to go in." What I did not know was that he'd just discovered that in actuality, our rental car was completely blocked in behind the other wedding guests.

I swallowed, to make sure my airway was clear enough. It was. I swallowed again. The reaction was on the wane, and the last thing I wanted to do was sit in a Roman ER for half the night, in formal wear, so they could tell me what I already knew.

"I'll be okay," I said. "Is the party over?"

The next day, we discovered the bigger problem. What pills I'd taken, plus a maintenance dose every four hours for the next day, exhausted the supply of Benadryl I had in my purse.

That was the only Benadryl I had packed. We would have to find more.

"You didn't pack any extra?" my mother asked. "Not one sheet?"

My mother tried her best to contain her irritation. At the age of twenty-one, I was only beginning to ease out of the hammock of my parents' care. I'd just assumed she'd packed a box, like always.

"Let's try Naples," my father suggested. "There's a military base there."

Though it was more than an hour out of our way, this seemed a sure bet. An American base would mean an American pharmacy. We made our way to Naples, my dad squinting over the steering wheel, trying to recall the way from his time spent posted in Italy thirty-some years before. My boyfriend rode shotgun, creasing and recreasing the map in hopes that somehow, the right fold would clarify our route.

What my dad did not know was that in the wake of the attacks in America on September 11, any references to the base had been scrubbed from public view, lest it become a target. We circled Naples over and over, each time veering into a seedier neighborhood.

"Can't we just ask someone?" I said, reaching to roll the window down. There was a group of young men sitting along the seawall, having a smoke. They looked like they could be sailors of some sort; maybe they would know where the base was.

"Do you have any idea where we are?" my father barked. "We are not stopping."

We came and left Naples without ever stepping outside the car. Instead, back in Rome, we found one of the kelly-green crosses that signified a *farmacia*, where we were directed to the shelf for sleep aids. Though it wasn't what we needed, at least those pills contained the active ingredient of diphenhydramine. I had no other option.

I would manage the rest of that trip without needing to take another Benadryl. My reaction didn't keep us from ringing in the New Year on Rome's Spanish Steps, fireworks overhead, confetti and champagne corks raining down on us in the crowd. We still made it to Pompeii, Florence, and Venice. But could I have done it on my own? What would it have been like if I hadn't had someone to come find me on that couch at the Majestic?

Sometimes, a friend mentions a semester abroad he did in college, or the summer he backpacked through Amsterdam.

"I wish I'd done that," I'll say absentmindedly. "Why didn't I do that?"

Once home, I'll remember that those options were never on the table when the topic of travel came up. As far as my parents were concerned, a semester abroad was a risk I couldn't afford to take. I'd learned my lesson about packing my own Benadryl. But no matter how many boxes I crammed into my suitcase, and how explicit or strategic I was in my allergy disclosure, there would always be a chef's mistake, the skeptical waiter, a housemate's drunken slipup. It wasn't that they didn't believe in me; I took care of myself to the best of my ability. It was the rest of the world they didn't trust.

. . .

February of last year, when I'd announced I was headed to New Orleans for five days, everyone had a suggestion of what to try. Crepes, they said. Pralines. Beignets at Café du Monde.

"Go get a burger at Snug Harbor and listen to jazz," my friend Josh told me. "Best burger in New Orleans."

"See if Messina's is still there," advised Greg, "and if so, get a muffuletta."

Perhaps noting that I was going to New Orleans for a conference on food allergies would have been enough to remind them that none of these foods is an option for me. Some cities are meant to be explored one signature meal at a time, whether it be *boeuf bourguignon* in Paris or spaghetti carbonara in Rome. What if you can't do that?

Walking through New Orleans on a chilly night, I wondered just how much I was missing. The night before, I had gone to Bourbon House and ordered the oysters, on the recommendation of a local poet who swore they were the best in town, sourced locally from P & J Select. I'd sat at the bar, sipping an Abita Turbodog as I watched them shuck open shell after shell, my anticipation mounting.

What they brought me were a half dozen fleshy, bland blobs—notable only for their size, as big as my palm. This was what I'd been waiting for? I looked at the diners around me and noticed that what they were devouring were Oysters Rockefeller (baked and topped with parsley, cheese, and bread crumbs) and Fonseca (heavy cream, peppers, and ham). No wonder. These oysters weren't prized for their liquor or their delicacy. I was trying to judge a dish by the taste of the plate.

So here I was, back on Bourbon Street, considering whether I should skip the meal and head straight to a hot toddy at

Preservation Hall. The French Quarter seemed an apropos place to drink one's dinner. Stopping to let a train of Mardi Gras–bedazzled twenty-one-year-olds pass, I looked up at the sign above the restaurant to my left.

Galatoire's, it said in black curlicue script.

Galatoire's. I'd heard of it. Jean Galatoire, a French immigrant, founded the restaurant in 1897 and opened its doors at 209 Bourbon Street in 1905. Tennessee Williams had a regular corner table, and made it the setting of Blanche and Stella's meal early on in *A Streetcar Named Desire.* I tried to recall the type of food that made Galatoire's famous. Ah, yes. Creole cuisine: an amalgam of French, Portuguese, Spanish, Caribbean, Mediterranean, Indian, and African ingredients, with Native American cooks throwing corn and bay leaves into the pot for good measure. In other words, exactly the kind of menu my mother would warn me away from.

But I was here. I was hungry, and I was dying to have one good authentic New Orleans meal. I headed inside.

"Walk-in for one?" the hostess inquired brightly. I confirmed, not realizing my answer secured a spot in the bustling downstairs room, which is always seated first come, first served. She directed me to the bar until they freed up a table. I perched on a stool and ordered a martini. As the bartender skewered an olive, then two, I worried I'd just made my first mistake.

"Are those olives stuffed with blue cheese?" I asked.

"Oh, no." He shot me a slightly offended look. "They are stuffed with anchovies."

When in Rome. Besides, I didn't have an anchovy allergy. I took a sip and found the brininess of any good dirty martini, without the cloud of olive-jar slop-water used by so many bartenders in lieu of actual juice. Interesting. I'd heard of chicken hearts in tequila before, but never fish in gin.

Soon I was summoned to the downstairs dining room, where they had made a nook for me by pushing a table up against one of the support beams, catty-corner to a group of fourteen. Everywhere, brass glinted and mirrors gleamed. The walls vibrated with the contrast created between emerald green, gilded with fleur-de-lis, and the crisp white of wainscoting and trim. Conversations interwove with the clinking of forks against china, which filled the air being churned by rows of ceiling fans overhead.

I cracked open the leather-bound menu to find dish after dish, each with an elegant name and unelaborated ingredients. I bit my lip. For every type of seafood I recognized, there was an unfamiliar treatment. Meunière Amandine? What the heck was "Yvonne garnish"? The sauces I knew, I knew to be butter based. Hollandaise. Béarnaise. Even the poultry had been rendered unrecognizable: Chicken Bonne-Femme, Chicken Clemenceau, Chicken Créole, Chicken Financière, Chicken Saint-Pierre, Chicken Comet, Chicken Cupid, Chicken Donner, Chicken Blitzen, and so on.

A tuxedo-clad man appeared before me. He had pale skin, cropped brown hair, and a warm smile. He looked like the kind of guy you'd want taking your sister to prom.

"My name is Preston," he said. "I'll be your server this evening. I see you've got a drink there. Can I get you started with anything else?"

"Don't get scared," I said. "But just so you know, I've got to stay away from dairy and egg. I've got food allergies."

Though I'd just wiped out over half the menu, he did not

blink. Without the pretense of whatever given fancy name, he recommended the fish of the day, drum, sautéed with artichokes, mushrooms, and crab.

"You'll love it," he said. He asked about appetizers.

"Is there anything on the 'green salad with garlic'?" I asked.

"No," he said. "Just *lots* of garlic."

"That's okay," I said. "I've got other allergies—croutons, cucumbers—but I find it's best to mention only what's relevant to the kitchen. Otherwise it overwhelms them."

He nodded. "We'll take care of you," he promised, sweeping up my menu and sidling past a waiter en route with a tray of oysters.

I wanted to believe him. I lifted my glass for a long sip and—*oooh*—already, something I'd forgotten to ask. I called him back. Did the dressing have mustard? Of course it did. Dressing diverted. Oil requested. A waiter attempted to deliver a basket of puffy loaves of French bread, each the girth of a small football. I waved him away.

Ten minutes later, Preston returned with my salad, which sans dressing turned out to also be sans garlic. One slick and fragrant leaf, clinging to the far rim of the plate, was the only evidence of the intended preparation. He looked down at me.

"That's the saddest thing I've ever seen," he said. I moved my hand defensively to my book: just another girl reading to distract herself from a dinner alone. Then I realized he was commenting on my empty martini glass. "What would you like to drink next?"

I asked him to pair a wine with the fish, and he suggested a Spanish white. My mind flashing back to the range of prices on the menu, I hesitated.

"It's not going to break a poet's budget, is it?" I asked.

"I wouldn't do that to you," he said. "It's one of the least expensive—seven dollars, I think—but if you like, I—"

"Never mind," I cut him off, blushing. "I trust you."

The greens were plain but crisp and sweet, and as I munched them I took in the choreography of service around me. The room was ringed in hooks, in part reflecting the dress code, which required jackets for men, and in part to clear whatever space possible between the densely grouped tables. If anyone had dared lay a coat over the back of a chair, it would have been swept to the floor by one of the ten waiters perpetually hustling over the black-and-white-patterned tiling. Every time the water level of my glass (helpfully labeled *Galatoire's*) threatened to sink below the halfway point, someone stopped what he was doing to dash over and fill it. Sometimes, as they edged past each other, one placed a protective hand on the small of another's back to guide him clear of a diner's jutting elbow. Other times they'd clasp and squeeze palms as they passed.

Preston returned, and with an elaborate twist of his wrist he swung a plate down.

"Here we have it," he said. "Drum, in a brown butter sauce."

I looked up at him. "Brown butter. Um. Dairy?"

"I will be *right* back," he said, whisking the plate away.

I was glad to have more time for people-watching. If ever one needed to argue that eating is as much a social ritual as a survival imperative, the proof is at Galatoire's. I could see why the line for their Friday lunch seating, which apparently winds down Bourbon Street, begins to form as early as 8 a.m. (Though regular patrons have the right to call in a proxy place-holder, no one gets to cut. Part of the house lore concerns the time Louisiana senator J. Bennett Johnston stepped out of line and into the restaurant in order to take a call inside from then president Ronald Reagan. When their conversation was over, he left the restaurant to get right back in line.)

All around me people were hopping tables, kissing cheeks, raising glasses. I tried to fill in the gaps to their stories. Surely the slight, happy blonde at the biggest table was celebrating her sixteenth birthday; surely that was her mother, the hair dyed a more silvery blond, her fingers twisting the pearls at her throat over and over. Surely the gray-haired foursome behind me, who had just erupted in applause as their waiter set fire to their bowl of Café Brulot, were seeing one another for the first time in twenty years. This was a fun game. Surely the gentleman in the seersucker suit, who had just slugged through his third Manhattan, was one of New Orleans's most prominent judges. Surely that was his longtime mistress in the pink cocktail dress and lacy shawl.

Preston returned and set down my plate once more. This time it was bare of any sauce, revealing instead the plate's concentric rings of green that set off a flourished proclamation: *Galatoire's*. Centered on the plate was a whole filet of drum, tucked beneath a tower of silky mushrooms, slabs of artichoke heart that had never seen the inside of a jar, and lumps of fresh crabmeat.

"Oh my," I said. "Thank you."

"You enjoy," Preston said, bowing his head slightly as he stepped away.

Each bite began with the moist drum, then yielded to the meatier artichoke and savory mushroom, before finishing with a top note of pure crab. Later, in consultation with the official Galatoire's cookbook, I'd figure out this was the menu's "Yvonne garnish" that I'd wondered about—in my case, minus the butter. The dish honored Yvonne Galatoire Wynne, daughter of Justin Galatoire, nephew of Jean himself. Preston hadn't just accommodated; he'd figured out a way to treat me to a house specialty.

As my tongue teased at the feathery bits of crab, I knew this was the kind of meal that could never be reduced to a series of recipes. It was the culmination of the room, the history, the service, and the cheerful din. The pleasure of each bite was intensified by the risk of trusting an unfamiliar city to take care of me, even when I was traveling alone. The taste was New Orleans.

When Preston brought my coffee, it took all my restraint to not slip the spoon into my purse as a trophy. *Galatoire's,* it said on the stem, in that now familiar script.

CHAPTER NINE

What Doctors Really Think

On the cusp of my thirtieth birthday, I had traveled to New Orleans to attend the annual conference of the American Academy of Allergy, Asthma, and Immunology (AAAAI). I know about food allergies from the ground up, based on firsthand experience. I wanted to hear what was being said from the top down. I wanted to know what doctors say about future treatments for allergies when their patients aren't around.

Though I know it's a licensed job, I've always thought of doctors in terms of personal relationships. My grandfather, my uncle, the allergist who has handled my case since I was one— all have cared for me with a mix of professional acuity and protective affection. My first serious boyfriend knew, even in high school, that he would become a doctor. I used to periodically check on the price of monogramming a stethoscope, thinking I would get him one as a graduation gift someday.

Though we broke up before he headed off to medical school, years later we'd still get together for the occasional awkward drink. One night he surprised me by mentioning that he might go into ear, nose, and throat medicine. I'd always imagined him as one of those superstars who finds a cure for cancer. He had assisted at a local university's oncology lab our senior year of high school. Who trades that in for hay fever and swimmer's ear?

"There's a lot of research to be done," he'd said, sipping his pint of Harp.

I kind of hated that he was now someone who drank beer. I kind of hated that I was now someone who drank beer. Our high school dates had consisted of walking down to the Wendy's two blocks from campus, where I'd order a Barq's root beer and French fries. We'd sit down at one of those tables that wobbled no matter how many yellow napkins you stuffed under the base, and I'd play the soda's squeaky-straw trombone as we talked. He'd take the first bite of his mayo chicken sandwich, and I'd remind him that there was no kissing from there on out. He'd stab the air with a fry for emphasis as he predicted a treatment for food allergies that worked, really worked. *It's a matter of time.*

Sitting in a downtown bar years later, on that awkward not-date, I was reminded of what had changed between us—and what had stayed exactly the same. "Ear, nose, and throat" is the umbrella for studies of asthma and allergy. Maybe there was a small part of him that still dreamed of fixing me. Maybe there was a small part of me that still dreamed of proving fixable.

But ROTC would take my ex on a detour through Japan, where he was assigned several years of service as a naval flight surgeon. All of my other doctor friends had gone into pediatrics. I arrived at the AAAAI conference with a schedule, an orange-ribboned press pass, and no tour guide. I'd have to make my way on my own.

Early on the first morning, I headed down to the Poster Session, where mobile "walls" had been built out of upholstered panels, creating aisles where abstracts presented throughout the conference were printed out and pushpinned up. Each poster measured as large as three feet eight inches high and seven feet six inches wide—eighth-grade science fair posters on steroids—and each row had a different theme, from "Asthma, Education, and the Underserved" to "Cytokines and Chemokines" to "IgE and Allergy." Some studies took an intuitive hypothesis—e.g., kids in the inner city are more susceptible to asthma—and saddled the sociological observation with data, percentages, and charts. Some studies were pure jargon unless you knew the relevant compounds by heart.

I made my way to the row marked FOOD ALLERGY I. The crowd surged in unpredictable waves, as people tried to talk to the exhibitors standing in front of their posters. Exhibitors periodically broke away and zigzagged down the row to talk to one another. It was as if I'd walked into a reunion for a college I had never attended. I didn't have the icebreaker of an institutional affiliation or the wingman of a colleague. I didn't recognize a single face.

Yet, in some ways, I felt completely at home. Maybe not with the allergists, but certainly with the allergies themselves. It was as if the posters in this row had been curated by the director of that old documentary series *This Is Your Life.* Every five feet, I found an answer to a question that had nagged at me. One poster outlined the difference in "restrictive" versus "permissive" diagnostic criteria for anaphylaxis. One poster documented reactions to soy among those with birch allergies. A quartet of posters discussed the allergenicity of baked milk versus raw. Pending publication in a peer-reviewed journal, all these abstracts were considered "preliminary findings." Still, if you wanted a portrait of where the science was heading, this was it.

Ninety-nine times out of a hundred, I am the only person in the room thinking about food allergies. In this place, I was surrounded by people who not only thought about food allergies but also dedicated substantive portions of their careers to the topic. From Arkansas to the Netherlands, from Tokyo to Cork, from Mount Sinai to Manitoba, center after center had sponsored these studies. It was both thrilling and deeply intimidating. I'd gone from being the default expert to the de facto rube.

I walked up the row, then back, then up again, until I realized it looked like I was pacing. I stopped in front of a University of Michigan poster on "the administration of influenza vaccine to egg-allergic children under thirty-six months." To this day, I've never taken a flu shot, based on the principle that it carries proteins from the egg in which the vaccine's ingredients are incubated. In flat, unemotional language, the abstract made clear that this was probably an outdated precaution.

As I struggled to reconcile ten seconds of reading with almost thirty years of my mother's prevailing wisdom on flu shots, a tall man with dark brown hair and a thin nose approached the poster's presenter. Though his suit was unremarkable, he had a sharp bearing; the woman from the University of Michigan straightened up as she answered his quick questions about their methodology and sample size. As he turned to go, I impulsively reached out and touched his shoulder.

"Yes?"

"I wanted to ask if—" If what? I had no plan. I tried to scan his name tag and hit a traffic jam of initials: F, A, A, A, A, I.

"—to ask if you were with the . . . Food Allergy and Anaphylaxis Network?"

That was the only organization that I could think to name, but as soon as I said it, I knew I was wrong. The acronym had not enough *A*s, no *N*s. His mouth pursed slightly.

"No," he said. "No, I'm with Duke."

Mistaking a university-sponsored allergy researcher for a FAAN staffer, in a setting like this, is akin to being on the Hill and mistaking a South Carolina Senator for a lobbyist. Not inconceivable but not really forgivable, either. He walked away and, fifteen feet down from where I stood, took up residence with his team. They were presenting not one but a whole constellation of posters, each bearing the logo of a shield, each toned in that distinctive Devil-blue palette. I watched as passerby after passerby stopped to give him a respectful nod and handshake.

Well. That was an auspicious start.

· · ·

Outside the medical community, the question everyone wants answered is, Why is the incidence of food allergy growing at such an alarming rate?

There are a handful of popular ideas, the most prominent of which is the Hygiene Hypothesis. The Hygiene Hypothesis suggests that in cultures where people are no longer routinely exposed to as many parasites, bacteria, and viruses as their ancestors, restless immune systems have turned their attention to harmless food proteins. Usually, this hypothesis surfaces as part of a larger nostalgic position that kids today are overprotected and missing out by not "playing in the dirt" more often.

There's even an experimental treatment specific to this theory, Helminth therapy, which posits that circulating small amounts of a parasitic worm ova (*Trichuris suis*, pig whipworm) through the body will desensitize those with food allergies. The effects of the residency of the worm itself are benign; the point is to give the immune system another target. Patients mix a vial of the ova with water or juice and drink it. Given that in recent years the breakfast industry has marketed every imaginable variety of orange juice—no pulp, extra pulp, calcium added, homestyle, pineapple blend—if this Helminth experiment proves fruitful, I'm looking forward to the "Now with an infusion of whipworm" campaign.

Though it is intuitively appealing, the Hygiene Hypothesis falters under logical scrutiny. The theory might justify why food allergy has surged in developed countries more so than in undeveloped countries. But why would incidence spike in inner-city settings, not rural environments? New York City basements and alleys don't lack for dirt.

Another hypothesis aims an accusing finger at the uptake of folic acid by pregnant women, who are hoping to ward off other birth defects. There's no purported mechanism of causation in place, but some find it a compelling concurrence that the 1980s saw both the rise of folate supplements and the rise of allergies in children.

Alternately, some point toward the correlation between vitamin D deficiency and skyrocketing rates of asthma, dermatitis, and allergy. I find it a stretch that low vitamin D levels would foster asthma, and not the other way around. After experiencing a few attacks, the kid with the inhaler is rarely the one rushing out to play kickball in the sunshine. And yes, the mother of a kid with eczema is going to slather him in sunscreen.

Within the world of allergists, the question of "why is this happening?" is moot in the short-term. The phenotypes of allergy sufferers are too diverse to draw meaningful conclusions based on contributing factors of lifestyle or ethnicity. Within the world of allergy research, the focus is on treating existing food allergies. That's where the suffering is palpable, and that's also where the money is. As Michael Pollan has argued, groups pursuing research often have to accept partial sponsorship for their clinics from those who profit from management, not prevention.

Most doctors believe desensitization is the key to treatment. For many years, allergic rhinitis has been predominantly treated by allergen-based injections. But there is another way. Injections were actually preceded—as early as 1905, in Germany—by experiments in administering minute dosages of allergens via droplets under the tongue.

Around 1910, New York pediatrician Oscar M. Schloss took on the case of a child, age two, with suspected egg allergy. His mother had noticed that when her son played with empty eggshells, hives broke out on his hands and arms. At the age of fourteen months, the boy had also exhibited extreme hives around the tongue and mouth after being given a soft-boiled egg to eat. That was the first egg the boy had ingested since a preliminary exposure at the age of ten days, when a bout of diarrhea had been treated with barley water and raw egg white. This was a common folk-cure of the time; barley water is still used today, minus the raw egg.

Schloss tested for allergy by injecting a guinea pig with the boy's blood, then feeding egg to the guinea pig. The guinea pig, which had previously tolerated egg, responded with symptoms of shock.

Schloss decided to treat the boy by mixing water with the white of a raw egg, diluting it over and over, and then finally feeding it to him. No reaction. The next day, he administered the same "medicine," diluting it a little less. No reaction. He did this the next day, and the next, each time making the solution stronger, until the boy could eat eggs in moderation. In 1912, he published the results of his treatment, suggesting that oral desensitization was a reliable option. But the enthusiasm for hypodermic treatment, as pioneered by Leonard Noon and John Freeman, had taken a firm hold on the market the year before, and would remain the dominant mode throughout the twentieth century.

The notion of taking treatments by mouth has been resurrected today under the terms sublingual immunotherapy (SLIT) and oral immunotherapy (OIT). With SLIT, a solution is deposited and held for one to two minutes under the tongue. The optimal frequency and duration of treatment has yet to be determined. SLIT offers the advantage of requiring only the tiniest amount of allergen, which, because it is internalized without going through the gut-based process of digestion and absorption, combines efficacy with an exceptionally low risk of anaphylaxis.

The SLIT method of treatment has been overshadowed by its younger brother, oral immunotherapy. In OIT, substantive milligrams of an allergen are ground up or otherwise reduced, combined with another food substance, and ingested daily in increasing amounts. Side effects, which are essentially minor reactions, tend to be limited to sneezing, nausea, hives, and vomiting—not bronchial distress—though there is a higher risk of anaphylaxis than with SLIT treatment. Doctors seem to prefer it as a technique, perhaps because it is mimetic of everyday eating, and they can envision a more natural transition from in-office to at-home treatment.

Most OIT treatments are paced over a matter of months if not years. But there has been preliminary investigation into "rush oral immunotherapy" (ROIT), which accelerates exposure by doubling the dosage each time (unless there is anaphylactic reaction) and administering it multiple times over the course of two weeks or less.

The second morning of the AAAAI conference, I was invited to attend a press forum on the latest developments in treatment for food allergies. I picked up a cup of sour (but free) coffee en route to grabbing my seat. We were being given audience with three top allergists, which could literally be referred to as the "A team": Hugh A. Sampson, Robert A. Wood, and A. Wesley Burks. They were experts I had seen quoted in article after article, without ever knowing the faces behind the names. One by one, they were introduced.

Dr. Hugh Sampson, of Mount Sinai School of Medicine in

New York City: spectacled, straightforward, hair slicing a quadratic curve across his forehead.

Dr. Robert Wood, of Johns Hopkins Children's Center in Baltimore: A shock of Santa-worthy white hair and, again, delicate eyeglasses. The word *disarming* comes to mind. This is, after all, the man who wrote *Food Allergies for Dummies*.

Dr. Wesley Burks: That thin nose. That expression, both mild and grave. Oh. Oh! Apparently I had met Dr. Burks, aka chief of the Pediatric Allergy and Immunology Division at Duke University, aka one of the world's top five experts in food hypersensitivity, the day before. When I mistook him for some guy from FAAN.

I hoped he did not remember me.

The AAAAI organizers had assembled this panel to discuss, in part, the latest results from a number of OIT experiments (and, to a lesser extent, SLIT experiments) being conducted across the country. The lead story concerned a trial headed by Dr. Burks, coordinated between Duke University and the University of Arkansas for Medical Sciences, in which oral immunotherapy treatment appeared to increase the threshold levels (the amount of allergen that can be ingested sans reaction) among a group of peanut-allergic children.

The children who had received OIT, versus placebo treatment, expanded their thresholds from 315 milligrams, a fraction of a peanut, to 5,000 milligrams—approximately fifteen peanuts. In another set of just-released experimental results, fifty-five egg-allergic children between the ages of five and eighteen had been randomized to receive OIT, using either egg whites or a placebo. In subsequent food challenges given forty-four weeks into OIT treatment, more than half of the forty who received

OIT egg whites "passed" by ingesting egg without reaction; not one did from the control group. Taken together, these studies were a testament to the potentials of OIT.

These are the kinds of experimental outcomes that, by the time they land in *USA Today* or the *New York Times,* are wrongfully portrayed as promising a cure for allergy. The news stories are often illustrated by a stock photo of a smiling child at the lunch table. Because the media doesn't measure success in milligrams, they round up to the nearest breakthrough even if it is at the cost of accuracy. The questions become, Can they eat scrambled eggs for breakfast yet? What about a peanut butter sandwich?

Reporters are not the only ones quick to hop to the lily pad of a cure. Doctors, facing constant queries from parents, are anxious for these trials to yield a practical course of treatment—one covered by health insurance.

"Everyone in the medical community asks, 'Can I take this back to my office now?'" Dr. Wood told us.

But as the doctors at the heart of the research were quick to caution, we are not there yet. Not by a long shot. OIT has to be recalibrated every time the patient suffers breathing distress, and any number of things outside the doctor's control can derail treatment, from viral infection to exercising too soon after exposure.

One of the biggest gaps between what the media reports and what researchers deliberate over is the gap between *desensitization* and *tolerance*. There is accumulating evidence for the ability to induce desensitization, in which allergens do not cause reactions as part of a steady, ongoing exposure trial. But we are only just beginning to test the ability to maintain tolerance, in which the subject can digest an allergen safely in the absence of supervised treatment.

In other words, as doctors ask among themselves, What happens when the oral immunotherapy stops? Will the child resensitize? Need there be an artificial supplement, a daily pill like a vitamin, that guarantees allergen exposure?

In addition to the study that desensitized children to peanuts, Duke and the University of Arkansas staged a study that looked at establishing residual tolerance. Twelve children who completed between thirty-two and sixty-one months of OIT, to the point of being considered desensitized to the allergen, were retested with an oral food challenge four weeks after going off treatment. Nine of the twelve subjects passed.

On one hand, that's great that nine children could then add peanuts to their diets. On the other hand, that's a 25 percent rate of relapse. For three families, all the progress earned with years of time-consuming and nerve-racking treatment unraveled in one month. Even for those who didn't relapse after one month, what is to say that they won't relapse after three months, or six?

"None of us—and each of us sees food allergy patients—" Dr. Burks said, looking at his colleagues. "None of us would practice this now."

Scientists are also looking at the difference in reaction levels among allergic children to "baked" variations on food, in which the food's protein has been heated or denatured. The key is epitope diversity. An IgE antibody reaction is triggered by the antibody's recognition of a site on the allergen molecule— an epitope—that matches the IgE's target pattern. Because this epitope is rendered in three dimensions, it may appear as designed, with the amino acids in sequence (the "sequential epitope"), or it may be altered, folded over itself so that nonadjacent acids are juxtaposed and seem as if they are in sequence (a "conformational epitope").

When a food is prepared—microwaved, sautéed, creamed, hydrolyzed, roasted, and so on—each process renders a conformational epitope. A child with limited epitope recognition who eats the food in one of these variant forms might fool her IgE antibodies into overlooking it. A child with diverse epitope recognition reacts regardless.

Figuring out the role of epitopes has helped explain some of the quirkier mysteries of food allergies. Take allergies to shellfish, historically one of the most troubling and persistent of the "big eight." It turns out that those allergic to shellfish typically have especially diverse epitope recognition: they are primed to recognize traces of shellfish in any form, whether raw or cooked or reduced to its broth.

Or look at nuts. One of the reasons there is so much overlap within the sphere of nut allergies is that the epitope patterns are so similar. A person with walnut allergy might react to a macadamia protein not because she is allergic to macadamia but because her body mistakenly reads the epitope as being from walnut. Some scientists wonder if the rise of peanut allergies is related to the fact that most commercially available peanut butter has become hydrogenated, which changes its prevalent epitope shape. In stabilizing peanuts for the sake of storing them in a jar, we may have destabilized their consistent ability to be recognized as food by the body. The body attacks what it does not see as nourishment.

On a pragmatic level, doctors are relieved to find a justification for many of the troubling contradictions they hear while taking case histories. "All of us have, in the past, had mothers come in and report that the child 'tolerated a cupcake,'" Dr. Sampson said. "Doctors were uncomfortable with that—we weren't thinking about it in terms of the structural molecular shift." The mothers weren't crazy. In some cases children reacted to raw milk only. Baked milk snuck past their immune systems.

Sitting in the audience, I had to keep reminding myself that this was a press conference, not storytelling hour. I craved the chance to share my firsthand experience. Despite having a confirmed egg allergy, for years I ate tempura on occasions when well-meaning waitresses assured my parents there was no egg. They thought we were asking about fresh egg, I'm sure. They didn't think about batters with dried, premixed ingredients. While some of the tempura batters might have been a Westernized quick-fry of flour, as I learned more about traditional Japanese cuisine, I became certain there was more than one occasion when I was exposed to egg. But the allergen was in such a thoroughly denatured form, its epitope such a weird variation on its natural shape, that I did not react.

Once I wised up, I couldn't enjoy tempura anymore. Yet by then I was into sushi, and I would order the occasional sushi roll with imitation crab or spicy tuna. Eventually I figured out that these, too, probably contained small amounts of egg. Why hadn't I ever reacted? I had always been too embarrassed to ask Dr. Latkin, my allergist, expecting to be chided for even risking an allergy attack.

I wish I had that kind of occasional tolerance when it came to dairy. Many do. A 2008 survey published in the *Journal of*

Allergy and Clinical Immunology estimated that 75 percent of the children living with cow's-milk allergy could tolerate extensively heated milk. As the panel pointed out, this is an extremely encouraging statistic for two reasons: One, it has potency as a predictor for those who may outgrow their allergy. Two, it means that if these children undergo OIT, there is a form of the allergen that can be administered with reasonable confidence that anaphylactic reaction will not occur.

Dr. Sampson led the research team behind the 2008 baked-milk study. His hope is to develop a blood-assay test that can dentify the baked-milk-tolerant majority, who can then adopt an allergy management plan that—instead of preaching 100 percent avoidance—includes some common dairy-containing foods.

But as he told the audience, his team is struggling with the fact that not all baked-milk products are alike. They had begun by challenging patients with muffins and waffles, with consistent success. Yet when they switched to using pizza ("because that's what everyone wanted," he said), 15 percent of those who could tolerate a muffin could not tolerate pizza. The problem was probably that the cheese offered an overly concentrated exposure to casein. The next goal was to see if puddings could be deemed safe—which would be a boon to parents everywhere trying to pack school lunches for an allergic child. But puddings, which combine a high dairy concentration with a low cooking temperature, have proven particularly difficult.

As I listened to these doctors talk more about immunotherapy options, I realized that—beyond a little good fortune with baked egg—I was a clinical terror. So many of these preliminary success stories include a preface, early on, of potential subjects who had been excluded because they would be "poor candidates" for further treatment. Those candidates typically had especially elevated IgE levels (like me) or a tendency to react to a particularly diverse range of allergen epitopes (like me) or multiple allergies (like me).

Will there be a division, a generation from now, between those with "treatable" and "chronic" food allergies?

One recent survey of six hundred charts from the Jaffe Food Allergy Institute showed that 78 percent of allergy patients between the ages of four and eighteen are avoiding an average of three to four allergens. Even if you discount those avoiding foods out of mere phobia, this suggests pediatricians are, by and large, treating patients with multiple allergies. What are the treatment options for those with more than one severe food allergy?

"That's where the Chinese medicine approach comes in," said Dr. Sampson.

Along with a colleague, Dr. Sampson has developed what is being called the Food Allergy Herbal Formula–2 (FAHF-2), currently under review by the FDA. This formula draws on centuries of practice by Chinese physicians, who have traditionally treated illness with herbs such as Qu Mai (*Dianthus superbus*), known for its pink flowers and its power to "move the blood." FAHF-2 combines nine herbs and would be administered in tablet form; upon ingestion, the herbs appear to release compounds that bind with IgE to the point of preventing anaphylaxis. Because it is not allergen specific, the formula has the potential to quell reactions even in a patient with multiple allergies.

Treatment with FAHF-2 is unlikely to prove tantamount

to a cure. But it might decrease sensitivity in a patient, like me, with perpetually and particularly elevated IgE levels. I could accept my allergies in terms of continuing to limit my diet but be able to live without fear of anaphylaxis from accidental allergen contamination. Or I could have the option of safely pursuing additional OIT or SLIT.

With the same purpose, some allergy patients have been experimentally treated with the anti-IgE monoclonal antibody omalizumab (known by its trade name, Xolair). Xolair is usually given to those with persistent and life-threatening asthma that has proven resistant even to high dosages of corticosteroids. But the cost of this drug, which was developed using recombinant DNA technology and appears to require a lifelong course of treatment, is exceptionally high—ten to thirty thousand dollars per year—not to mention that its long-term effects are unknown.

I remember going to my doctor years ago, when my mother had heard about "anti-IgE medicine" on the news. She'd wondered if it was something I should pursue.

"The thing is, your body is *supposed* to release IgE in response to a lot of things," my skeptical HMO internist told me. "Think of those treatments as a broadsword. What you need is a scalpel." One of the advantages of Chinese herbs over Xolair, besides cost, is their record of use in folk medicine. We have the reassurance that generations have ingested them without causing internal catastrophe.

Would I try the Chinese herbal treatment, if and when the pills are in general circulation? I don't know. When I will later mention it to my mother, upon return to D.C., she will bristle instinctively against the risk. "You couldn't try *all* nine herbs at once," she will caution. "What if you react to any one of them the same way you do to mustard?"

The panel wrapped up, and I hung back as reporters swarmed the three doctors. Though I wanted to talk to them, I wasn't sure what I had to say anymore. I wanted to applaud their research, yet I kept thinking about the high stakes and low yield of these therapy techniques. I tried to wrap my head around how many cycles of testing, peer review, and government approval would have to take place before the general food-allergic population sees OIT as an option in their local allergist's office. From a reporter's perspective, solving the problems of one allergic kid heralds "a cure." From a patient's perspective, our success stories are just beginning to be counted in the double digits, out of the millions affected.

Part of what hinders research is that few people want to volunteer their kids as guinea pigs. We're early enough in the allergic-population boom that there are not that many peanut-allergic adults available for testing yet, though that may change in a decade. Besides, when trying to fight a disease that can present differently (and more severely) in childhood, adult subjects alone are not an effective predictor of treatment potentials.

There are some experiments where animal subjects are useful. Standard laboratory mice have been made "allergic" to peanuts and egg by feeding the mice with a combination of allergen protein and enterotoxin. An enterotoxin is a toxin associated with gastrointestinal distress—such as staphylococcal enterotoxin B, which is linked to food poisoning, or the cholera toxin. The mice's resulting immunological response resembles that of an allergic reaction, because they increase production of white blood cells related to mediating airway inflammation. There appears to be an enduring allergic sensitization.

Then what? *You* try placing a droplet under that little mouse's tongue, much less ask Stuart Little if his throat itches. Let's face it: in a field where self-reporting of symptoms is critical, there's only so much you can do with a mouse.

A parent's decision to enter his or her child in a clinical trial has to weigh many factors. For some families there is a financial incentive—an opportunity to have scratch tests and RAST tests performed for free, not to mention the potential benefits of the experimental treatment. For most, it comes down to where they balance on the seesaw between optimism and frustration.

Riding down the escalator of the convention center, I overheard two allergists commiserating over their lack of experimental samples.

"We needed soy. But soy is impossible to get."

"I wish I'd known! I had a dozen soy, then sent them on out to California. Are you looking for egg?"

How odd to be spoken of not as a person but as a vial of allergic blood. I am *Soy.* I am *Egg, Cow's Milk, Tree Nut.* A few soft approaches were made to my parents, when I was young, suggesting that we might take part in the studies being mounted at Johns Hopkins, just an hour up Route 95. We shrugged it off. I'm not a good donor; my veins are hard to find, easily bruised. I didn't want to spend my summer as a lab rat.

Now part of me wanted to lean forward, tap one of those doctors on the shoulder, and offer up my arm for the draw. Which would have been, to use professional parlance, "a really freaky thing to do." So I did nothing.

Later that night, back in the hotel room, I pored over the materials I had picked up during the day. In the Fall/Winter 2009 issue for a newsletter called *Support Net*, I found an article by journalist Beth Puliti that profiled the experiences of three mothers whose children agreed to take part in experimental studies.

Puliti wrote about one parent, Joy Hogge, Ph.D., who hoped her nine-year-old son might build up a tolerance to peanuts. But in the double-blind study, his dose of applesauce mixed with powdered substance (peanut, though the "blind" doctors didn't know that) resulted in an anaphylactic reaction that raged through a shot of epinephrine, several Benadryl, three days' worth of steroids, and an oxygen mask.

Hogge was amazed when, one month later, he agreed to a second attempt at desensitization. Several weeks into treatment, his threshold had hit a plateau of 12 milligrams. He struggled with stomachaches, itchy throat, and asthma-like attacks.

"These symptoms, along with his memories of the challenge and the fact that he learned he hated the taste of peanut, were very hard for him," Hogge told Puliti. "He decided to discontinue the study."

I put aside the article to reread it more thoroughly once I was back at home. Later, it clicks: Arkansas. The trial's only identifier is its location, Arkansas Children's Hospital in Little Rock.

At the press panel, we had all been inspired by hearing about the twenty-three children who were taking part in the oral immunotherapy treatment for peanut administered by Duke and . . . the University of Arkansas for Medical Sciences, which partners with ACH. Fifteen children who had received OIT treatment all along (eight had received placebo) had already experienced increased desensitization, the ability to eat those precious fifteen peanuts without reaction. But looking at the parameters of the abstract, I realize that *twenty-nine* subjects were originally enrolled. Six did not make it to the oral food challenge stage. Had Hogge's son been among the six?

There must have been a moment when the doctors running the trial said, among themselves, "This kid is not going to be desensitized." Then they may very well have said to the mother, "It's up to your family." And perhaps she had said to her son, "It's up to you."

I'd thought that parsing out these gaps between what is said and what is believed would be revealing, even strategic. But the gaps are simply a matter of human nature. These doctors are as hopeful as they can be and as helpful as they can be, but at the end of the day, they're human. It's a big relief. And frightening.

. . .

On my last day at the AAAAI conference, I walked through the exhibit hall. Laboratories, professional societies, advocacy groups, medical supply companies, and niche start-ups all jostled for the attention of the crowd. There wasn't much of a crowd to be jostled for—more a scattering of people here and there. With tightrope precision I stayed to the center of each aisle, to avoid outstretched hands offering brochure after brochure. Paper is the enemy of trying to travel with only a carry-on bag.

Occasionally a free sample would lure me to a vendor's table. I picked up a couple of packets of SunButter, a salty, oozy, oddly tasty spread made from sunflower seeds. If there can be a plus side to an epidemic, it might be the profusion of "butters" produced in the wake of peanut allergies.

I said hello to the folks from FAAN. I left a card for the people from the Food Allergy Initiative. I talked for a while to the woman who founded Kids With Food Allergies, which publishes the *Support Net* newsletter. Kids With Food Allergies is a Pennsylvania nonprofit that focuses on creating a network where families can share tips for coping with allergic conditions. We got on the subject of birthday cakes, and she told me that some parents are forgoing food-based treats entirely. Instead, the cakes were made of felt, decorated collaboratively by classmates as a gift to the birthday kid.

Each year, the AAAAI conference gives free exhibit space to a particularly deserving and urgent cause. This year's recipient was The Mastocytosis Society, dedicated to serving those with overactive mast cell populations, which means someone who is trapped in the perpetual state of inflammation and edema associated with allergic reactions. The TMS table workers had bright smiles, a pile of flyers, and high-end swag in the form of emblazoned flashlights. None of it did any good. The exhibition room was where people came to wander as they sipped their coffee or had a quick lunch, yet their display could not have been less appetizing. No one wants to stare at an oversized picture of a pustule-covered little girl as he eats a Thai chicken-salad wrap.

Far more popular were the megabooths sponsored by pharmaceutical companies. These booths, which were set off by their own swaths of carpet and stand-alone lighting, featured made-to-order kettle corn, free massages, and robots.

The star of the floor was an electronic creature sponsored by Asthmatx, Inc., as part of the publicity push for Asthmatx's Alair Bronchial Thermoplasty System. Sporting a plastic faux crewcut, yellow-lensed sunglasses, and the name VASO on its plastic-polymer clavicle, this eight-foot-tall creature bounced on two independently controlled feet as he took questions and cracked jokes with the audience.

"You think I was born this way?" he bragged, flexing. "I work out."

The robot's body was paneled in purple and blue, with a torso too slender for an actual person to hide inside. I'd heard about this technology before. Somewhere nearby there had to be an operator, seeing through cameras behind the robot's eyes, hearing through microphones planted where its ears would be, and wearing an exoskeleton of body sensors that translated every move in real time. The robotics industry calls them anthrobots.

Every few minutes, VASO would break out in dance in response to a prerecorded sound track. The track, every time, was the Bee Gees' "Stayin' Alive." No one else seemed to find this an odd choice to promote a breathing medication.

"You lookin' at me?" he asked. "You lookin' at me?"

I had reached my saturation point. Too many slogans. Too many business cards. Backing away from the Alair booth, I began navigating toward the exit.

Before I reached the double doors, another robot caught my eye. It was silver, about six feet tall, with big, blue bug eyes and a butler's posture, vaguely masculine. Its squat, wheeled base evoked Johnny 5 in *Short Circuit*.

I stepped closer, checking for the logo of the robot's sponsor.

Sanofi-aventis U.S., otherwise known as the makers of Allegra. I felt an unexpected surge of pride. I've been on Allegra for years. Claritin, Seldane, Zyrtec—all the other allergy medications used lactose-derivative binders that, after reaching a few weeks of critical mass in my bloodstream, had caused rashes to break out along my forearms. Only Allegra had proven safe. So I'd fought for it, even when several different HMO insurance plans had tried to switch me to generics or substitutes, and paid out of pocket at times. If this was a pennant race, I'd stumbled across the bleachers for my home team.

Should I go over? The robot, which had been making polite conversation with a woman in a navy skirt-suit, pulled a three-point turn to face me. We looked at each other.

"Hi, Sandra," he said.

I raised my hand in a half wave, confused by this familiarity. Then I remembered I was wearing a name tag. I looked around, sure I'd spot someone speaking into their wrist or lapel. But the voice behind the robot was well camouflaged.

"Hi," I said.

"Come closer," he said. "I won't bite."

I was tempted to step onto Allegra's carpeting. But I was conferenced out, and New Orleans was waiting.

"Next time," I said.

"I'll miss you," he replied. The bulbs behind his eyes blinked.

I put my fingers to my lips and blew a kiss to the robot. Then I turned and walked away, away from the convention center, away from the doctors. I did not look back.

CHAPTER TEN

The Nature of Nurture

Several years after our ill-fated Lemon Drop shot at Maarten's, Kristen was still my best friend, her now husband, Bob, was no longer a fireman, and Keira—their daughter—was approaching her first birthday. There was talk of cake. Not any old birthday cake, but a cake in the shape of a ladybug, spiked in pink and brown frosting (more appetizing than red and black), complete with Twizzler legs and antennae, and Hershey's Kisses pressed tip-down into the yellow cake to provide ladybug spots. In fact, make that two cakes. One for the party guests, and one custom-sized for Keira.

On the day of the celebration, I was running late—as always, underestimating the slog of traffic from my downtown D.C. apartment to their house in the suburbs. Every few minutes, I checked the clock, groaned, and patted the bright bag on the passenger seat. Maybe the set of mirrored, bejangled building blocks I'd bought as a gift would be my ticket to forgiveness.

When I finally walked in, more than an hour into the party, I wasn't surprised to find a full and well-decorated house. Somewhere in between hemming the dresses of her own bridesmaids and remodeling her kitchen from scratch, Kristen had become the Martha Stewart of our group of high school friends. (Not the saccharine Martha, either; the sarcastic, fun, post-penitentiary Martha.) The dining room table was arrayed with homemade punch, *1st Birthday* napkins, sandwiches, and skewers of chicken satay. I smiled, noticing every sauce and dressing was set on the side. Sandra-friendly.

"Hey there," Kristen said as I put my bags down. I hadn't fully adjusted to viewing Kristen in mom mode. I still saw the fourteen-year-old who painted daisies on her toenails with three different shades of polish. Today her nails were gunmetal silver, a yelp of freedom paired with an otherwise practical gray T-shirt, jeans, and bobbed hairstyle. She was leaning down to catch Keira, who lurched across the living room with the manic gait of a new walker. Keira let out a profound squawk of protest as Kristen scooped her up a few feet shy of reaching her destined play set.

"She's a little overwhelmed," Kristen said. "She had a low fever all morning. And it's a lot of people."

Keira's ladybug shoes matched her ladybug cakes. The ladybugs on her T-shirt were so cartoonishly round that they resembled polka dots, and I felt a wave of nostalgia. Just a few days earlier, my mother had reminded me that on my first birthday—the day when, as my mother always notes, I went in for my first allergy appointment—I had been wearing a pink-polka-dot dress.

Kristen sent one of her in-laws down to round up the men drinking beer in the basement, and I worried with a twinge that she had been waiting on my arrival to cut the cake. That was an exercise in futility, since I could not eat the cake, nor the Neapolitan ice cream, nor the individual chocolate crisps in their pink foil cups. But maybe Kristen knew I'd want to witness the big moment.

"Those are some amazing ladybugs," I told her.

"The black licorice turned out to be on the stale side," she said. "So that's for decoration only. Otherwise, so far, so good."

At every child's birthday party I have attended, the same truth emerges: a cranky one-year-old does not treasure being stuck in a high chair, surrounded by two dozen vaguely recognizable blobs of adulthood. Nor does she want a special hat, decorated with paper fringe, strapped onto her head with an elastic band. Nor does she want to be serenaded with "Happy Birthday." Yet this is what we did, because it is what is done at birthday parties. The crying erupted. The hat came off. Kristen offered up the ultimate birthday throne of a mama's lap, and finally—with Keira calmed down, and the offending licorice set to the side—we were ready for cake.

As the grown-ups passed around slices of the big ladybug, Keira stared at the tinfoil platter that held her mini version, dotted to scale with chocolate chips instead of Hershey's Kisses, and frosted with two wide eyes and a pink grin. Kristen placed a chunk of cake in the baby's grasp and waited. Instead of eating, Keira brought up the icing-rich fingers of her left hand to her face with a *Why me?* flourish. Gobs of pink soon coated her cheek, forehead, and hairline. She rubbed at her mouth, leaving behind streaks of what looked like dollar-store lipstick.

"Good thing you took photos beforehand," one of the guys said.

We kept waiting for Keira's triumphant bite of cake, but it never came. She just played with it. The women ate twice as enthusiastically, trying to make up for the birthday girl's apparent hunger strike. The men drifted back downstairs to where their beers were waiting. Kristen bounced Keira on her knees, then stood up and began pacing as the baby grew increasingly agitated, fussing again and again at her ears with her grimy fists. They went upstairs, we figured for a diaper change. When they came back down, I was surprised that she hadn't wiped the frosting off Keira's face.

"I think she's having an allergic reaction," Kristen said, looking at me. The pink on Keira's face wasn't frosting; it was hives that had come up underneath the frosting. This had never happened to her before. It wasn't only hives. Leaning in, Kristen had been able to hear her daughter wheezing for breath. One phone-call consult later, Bob and Kristen were getting ready to take Keira to the hospital. They draped her in a coat, rather than taking the time to work her arms through the sleeves, and scooted out into January's cold.

"It'll be fine," I'd said to them. "You go. We'll clean." It was a promise I meant but couldn't actually keep. The dining room table was covered in things I couldn't touch without breaking into hives of my own. Melted ice cream pooled on the dirty plates. I did a quick round of cup-and-napkin duty. Then I stood by helplessly as Bob's mother, sponge in hand, directed the clearing off, washing out, and stacking up.

"You're the one with all the allergies," one of Kristen's friends said to me. "What happened?"

"It had to have been the cake," I said. "But I know they've tried dairy before."

"Why does it have to have been the cake?" said Bob's mother. "She tried a lot of things today. It could have been the punch."

"Oh, I don't think so," I said, trying to choose my words carefully. "None of the fruits in the punch are common allergens."

"It had mango in it," she said.

"No it didn't," I said. I'd asked Kristen if it was safe, and she'd said it was. If it had had mango, I'd have been on the floor. (Later, she'd confirm: orange, pomegranate, ginger ale. No mango.) "Besides, it wasn't so much her mouth. The hives were on her face, where she'd spread the frosting. Maybe the food dye?"

"I don't know," Bob's mother said. "Jon had this reaction to shellfish once, and the hives showed up all over."

"Yeah, but hives in the exact same shape as the frosting? I bet it's the dye."

I wanted to be right about the icing, but not for the sake of contradicting Bob's mom. Not exclusively. Intolerance to Red Dye #40 seemed better than any of the alternatives of allergy to wheat, milk, or egg. But no matter what, a reaction of such intensity, with primarily topical exposure and at a young age, was a bad sign.

One hour, one IV, one round of Benadryl, one dose of steroids, and one pacifier later, Keira was almost back to normal. But her parents would soon learn that her version of normal includes an allergy to egg. This diagnosis would eventually broaden to include what their doctor called the "holy trifecta"—allergy, asthma, and eczema. Within a few months of changes in diet and nightly nebulizer treatments, their once often-fussy toddler had transformed into a happy, goofy little girl.

Given the statistics, I knew at least one of the children born to my friends was going to exhibit food allergies. I just wasn't expecting to be on hand for the big debut. On the way home from the party, I had called my mother and rehashed the whole debacle, right down to the polka-dot déjà vu.

"I felt like, somehow, with all my experience, I should have been able to *do* something," I told her. "There was nothing I could do."

"It's an awful feeling," my mother said. "I know."

At least Keira has come into a world where allergic reactions are recognized within minutes. I try to imagine what it must have been like for my mother, not knowing why I refused her breast, each bottle of milk and then Similac making me sicker. There is no bond that comes easier to mother and child than the act of cradling and feeding, except when what you're feeding your child is actually killing her.

In the weeks after Keira's birthday party, I found myself wondering what would happen when it was my turn. My mother had been unable to get me or my sister to breast-feed for any length of time. Could I convince my child to breast-feed? While there's plenty of anecdotal evidence that the predisposition toward food allergies is inherited, there's no model for specific allergies being passed down a family line. Odds are that my children will not share my allergy to cow's milk. If I can't breast-feed, how do I handle a bottle filled with something that could put me into anaphylactic shock? Every round of spit-up, every spill, is a recipe for disaster.

Later, when my children advance to solid foods, a whole other set of questions will come to the table. Do I limit my kids to my diet, for the sake of a safer household? How do I prepare them for the inevitable days when they make me sick? "Don't touch Mommy until you've washed up": that's got to be the prescription for a high-strung child.

One of my favorite movies is *Steel Magnolias.* It came out when I was nine, and I've probably seen it two dozen times, if not more. Part of my love is fueled by its strange caricatures of Southern culture: Drum hacking the ass off the armadillo groom's cake to reveal its bloodred interior, or Annelle solemnly informing Dolly Parton's character, "Miss Truvy, I promise that my personal tragedy will not interfere with my ability to do good hair."

There's also one scene that haunts me. Shelby, the character with diabetes played by Julia Roberts, collapses on her front porch while alone and caring for her young son, Jackson Jr. She goes to call for help and crumples again. Her husband comes home to find his son wailing, the spaghetti boiling over on the stove, and his wife sprawled on the steps, unconscious, her hand still clutching the phone receiver.

The scene is sentimental Oscar bait, I know. In the real world, tragedy can strike anyone, anytime—aneurysms, strokes—I know. But now, in my thirties, watching those around me begin their families and dreaming of my own, I realize that it's one thing for me to play the odds of this allergic life. It's another to bet the welfare of a child on them.

"You need to talk to my friend Jenny," Erika says when I confess what has been on my mind. "She's like you."

Erika isn't kidding. Jennifer Kronovet is only a few years older than me and lives with her husband, Anthony, and her son, Solomon. She is allergic to milk, tree nuts but not peanuts, and sesame seeds—not quite the variety of allergies that I have, but equal in their severity.

"I go into minor anaphylactic shock," she says with the casual tone I recognize from years of practice. "Even now, having learned to avoid those foods, things happen."

When her parents sent her to college, they packed a box of infant formula. She liked to eat cereal in the mornings, and before the age of rice-, almond-, and soymilk options, that was all she'd ever used to pour into her bowl. I'm the last person to judge her for this. After all, I was the one they called "fish girl."

The parallels mount up. When I was getting my birthday hazelnuts, Jennifer was being doled out one of her mother's homemade pumpkin muffins, invariably still frozen rock solid from the elementary school's freezer. She'd have to scrape at it with her teeth until it softened.

"We were trailblazers," she tells me. Jennifer found comfort, as I did, in having a close group of friends who got to know her allergies. Even today, when she comes over for dinner parties, everything is labeled. "This is the Jenny-safe spoon; this is *not* the Jenny-safe spoon," her hosts inform her.

"They joke, 'It's like we're keeping Jenny-kosher,'" she says.

Her son turned one in April 2010. He is not allergic to milk, and has not yet been tested for nuts or sesame. (Earlier that year, a widespread recall for manufacturing defects effectively cleared child and infant doses of Benadryl, along with Tylenol, Motrin, and Zyrtec, off the U.S. market. That derailed a lot of at-home allergy testing.) But after trying scrambled eggs, he broke out into hives. His oral food challenges with baked egg and egg yolks have gone smoothly, so they're going to try again with egg whites, which are often more allergenic because they contain a higher density of proteins than the yolks. Jennifer is hoping the first reaction will prove to have been a fluke.

"If he's going to have an allergy, it's so frustrating to have it not be the *same* allergy," she says.

Because her husband, Anthony, is lactose intolerant, their household as a young couple had been virtually dairy free. Then came Solomon.

"I wanted to cut back on our breast-feeding, but kids get used to drinking milk. Soy has issues because of the hormones," she says; some research indicates the phytoestrogens in soy and tofu may disrupt hormone balance in the body. "Rice milk is so sweet," she adds. With her options dwindling, Jennifer decided to give cow's milk a try.

She shares my fears about handling the dairy with her bare hands.

"I don't like touching it. But nothing has happened so far." Besides, there has been an unexpected therapeutic aspect to bringing milk into Sol's life. "Watching him eat dairy is so great for me. It's so much more wide-open for him—he's liberated."

In the interests of heading off any allergies that might form in the absence of exposure, her doctors advised Jennifer to "feed him what normal people eat."

"You have no idea how little I know about what normal people eat," Jennifer remembers thinking. "Do normal people eat bread with avocado for dinner every night? Because that's what I eat." She has no choice but to be brave.

"I just want him to be able to eat as many different things as he can. We've tried Ethiopian food. We've tried rabbit." She pauses. "For me, food has always been associated with fear and death. He takes so much pleasure in food."

"The only sad thing is that he wants to feed me," she continues. "'No, Mommy can't,' I have to tell him. We have a whole play-feeding thing now."

Jennifer has another friend who has given birth to a daughter severely sensitive to many things, including seeds and dairy. Mom has no allergies of her own. "She can eat off my plate, but not her mom's," Jennifer says of the baby they call "Jenny's baby," as if the stork dropped her off at the wrong address. "It's a whole new thing to her."

Like me, Jennifer wants to use her experience to help the next generation of allergic kids have an easier time. She tells people to use kosher guidelines to steer toward dairy-free desserts. She carries a translated note listing her allergies when she travels.

"I feel like I've accumulated a lot of tricks," she says. "So much focus on feeding kids is about health. But there's the social side, too. You need to tell them, if you're out with your friends at a café, just get the French fries. You'll be fine with fries."

I ask what her biggest concerns are when it comes to her son's diet.

"I'm more worried about him eating rocks and leaves and handfuls of dirt," she says. "When it comes to something he's allergic to, I know what's going to happen. But eating a piece of glass off the playground—who knows?"

Food allergies are daunting. Yet with kids, she says, she has come to feel "there's way worse things you're going to worry about." Her son is at an age when outgrowing his allergies is not only possible but likely. Yet if he still has his allergies when he is ten, or older, her perspective might change.

Another allergy mom who agreed to speak to me finds herself mulling over the future for her twelve-year-old daughter, who is allergic to tree nuts.

"I don't think she understands, at some level, how serious it can be," she comments, describing how one day her daughter lackadaisically mentioned a reaction to hazelnut. The teenage years loom large. "I hope someday she gets to kiss someone— but she'll need to consider what he ate beforehand."

Venturing into the world of alcohol won't be easy, either. You can never know what cutesy cocktail is hiding a dash of Frangelico or Amaretto. "It looks very pretty," she imagines having to warn her child, "but the umbrella doesn't make it safe."

In addition to sharing a tree-nut allergy with her daughter, her oldest, this woman is allergic to wheat (complicated by celiac disease), egg, and oranges. When she first got pregnant, she was determined to avoid passing along her problems.

"I stayed away from everything I was allergic to, plus all the other common allergens: shellfish, peanuts, et cetera," she tells me. "I had a spotless house. You've never seen anyone clean so much. Hardwood floors, no drapes. I made my husband replace the blinds so we had the ones that catch less dust."

"I either did everything I could," she says, with a laugh, "or else exactly the wrong thing." These days, doctors don't recommend these tactics.

For her next child, she did nothing out of the ordinary, and at age eight, he seems to have no allergies. Yet in his early years of school, he refused to eat oranges or drink juice at school. Why? He had figured out, on his own, that his contamination with citrus prevented him from being able to kiss his mother when he got off the bus.

She does not keep oranges in the house; just the odor, she says, is enough to nauseate her. Her husband is not crazy about the ban on orange juice. He can empathize with avoiding foods—he had allergies to dairy and tomatoes in childhood—but he outgrew them, retaining only a few quirky sensitivities.

"He can't touch escargot," she says. "The last time he did was fifteen years ago, and it was awful." So her husband is in charge of cooking eggs (hold the snails) for the kids in the mornings, using the same designated pan each time, which he cleans. She has asked him not to feed eggs at all to their youngest child, a one-year-old.

"I'm worried that if he's not cleaned up properly, and I kiss him ..." she lets the sentence trail off. "And he's not a neat eater. He's a messy eater."

It's strange to talk to someone who has a worse variation on one of "my" allergies. The virulence of her sensitivity to egg was brought home to them a few years back, when the family awakened one night to find a bat in the house—specifically, a bat tangled in her hair. Flailing caused it to attack rather than retreat, which is symptomatic of rabies; the bat fled to the attic before anyone could capture it for testing. So the whole family was subjected to rabies shots, which, like influenza vaccines, are cultured in egg.

"The first time was okay, the second time I felt sick, the third time I had breathing trouble," she tells me. "The fourth time, I had anaphylaxis. By the fifth shot they had to give me a special version, cultured in human immunoglobulin."

Unlike Dracula, wheat isn't known for dive-bombing its victims in the night. But it can feel like a bat in the attic in their house: a constant, hovering threat.

"I'm neurotic and obsessive about everyone washing their hands," she says.

I ask what the biggest challenge has been. "The struggle is not seeing myself in my kids," she answers. She has to remind herself that every report of a "bad feeling" is not proof of some new food allergy. Every day, kids get colds, tummy aches, fevers, not to mention cases of outright-faking-it.

"And yet I'm trying to be sensitive in a way my parents, out of ignorance, were not sensitive to me," she says. "My dad was of the mind that if you don't vomit every time you eat a sandwich, you're not really allergic to wheat." Apparently, he never got over his skepticism.

"He was a stockbroker," she says, "not a biologist."

On the upside, her father's refusal to recognize her condition meant she was allowed to do a lot more than most children with food allergies of such severity, including five-day trips to

YMCA camp. Now she sends her nut-allergic daughter off to camp with three weeks' worth of premade meals, which the counselors prepare using a separate pot and utensils, and two EpiPens.

I'm curious as to whether she's ever used her own EpiPen. I get asked this a lot, and my answer is "No, but there were plenty of times I should have." So I ask her.

"I would rather stay curled up in a ball, drink Benadryl until the cows come home, and miss life for twenty-four hours," she says, "than use an EpiPen."

"Why?"

"Honestly," she says, "I hate to admit that kind of weakness."

"Me, too," I say.

This is one of those things you're not supposed to say out loud. There is a legion of food-allergic adults out there who, year after year, buy epinephrine autoinjectors and, year after year, do everything in their power to avoid using them. At the end of the year, they expire. We buy them again. Again, we carry them everywhere. Again, we don't use them. Meanwhile we advocate for much more liberal use of EpiPens in schools. Recently, the mother of a nine-year-old with food allergies put me on the spot.

"Is it fear?" she questioned. "Does it hurt? What can I say to my daughter that would make her use her EpiPen?"

I tried to explain to her that the inhibitor isn't pain. A sting in the thigh is nothing when your throat is swelling shut. Maybe it's that Benadryl and breathing aids are largely self-metered. You can treat yourself—"miss life for twenty-four hours," so to speak—and come back with no one the wiser. Epinephrine tips that first domino in the line that leads to the hospital. Ambulance fees. Paperwork. IVs.

"But it's not the injection that is sending you to the hospital," my friend insisted. "It's the reaction."

"Let me be clear," I said. "I'm not claiming these are the right things to do. I'm just telling you why I do them."

I take this all back to my mother, wondering if she has a theory.

"It's a control thing," she says. "It runs in the family." Even an issue as serious as food allergies cannot trump our basic natures. She reminds me of the reaction I had when I was seven or eight, out with my parents and grandparents. On our way to an exhibit of ancient Chinese artifacts, we had gone to dinner at Hogate's, a local seafood place. Somehow my plate had been contaminated—maybe fried shrimp, maybe butter—and the roof of my mouth began itching. A few minutes into the car ride away from the restaurant, I had vaulted from the backseat into the front, so I could press my face against the air conditioner; a child's version of an oxygen mask.

"Your father knew how to get to George Washington Hospital," she remembers. "Then we sat forever in the waiting room."

This was when I had always remembered him telling me, *Breathe. Just breathe.* What I had forgotten was my grandfather the doctor, borrowing a nurse's stethoscope so he could take my vitals while we waited. My mother had called Dr. Latkin, my allergist, who prescribed steroids based on her report. My family essentially ran clinic out of the lobby. By the time they were ready to admit me, I was ready to go home.

"There was a risk to how we handled things," she says,

admitting that it is sometimes one she regrets in hindsight. "I remember that reaction in Nashville, or that one to pistachios. You could have died. But we didn't want you to grow up with hospitalization after hospitalization. And the way you are now, so independent—I do think it comes back to that, a little.

"At least," she adds, "I hope so."

For weeks I've been obsessing over the ways food allergies come between a parent and child. The rejection of breast milk; the anxiety of a mother trying to cook foods she would never touch for herself; the hesitation of a child who does not want to give his father hives with a kiss.

But I have to honor that there's an intimacy being created there, too, one unique to any parent who manages a child's chronic illness. My mother, the diplomat. My mother, the (un) registered nurse. My mother, the translator of cries and bubbles.

If my child did have allergies, I'd know where I'd look for guidance. My mother, the teacher. If kids like Jennifer and I had blazed a trail, it's only because parents like her cleared the path.

. . .

"When milk was twenty-six cents a quart, my parents paid seventy-five cents for goat's milk, and then had to boil it," a woman writes to me. *The Washington Post* had recently published a column I'd written about my dinner-party mango reaction, and she sent a letter describing her own experience with food allergies. Decades earlier, a prick test for sixty substances had caused numerous wheals to break out across her back. The doctor decreed that she could have no beef, pork, wheat, or cow's milk—and most vegetables were rationed to only once a week, to prevent overexposure.

"If I had tomato juice on Monday, I couldn't have stewed tomatoes until the next Monday," she remembers.

In an era when regular bread cost sixteen cents per loaf, they had struggled to pay almost a dollar each for loaves of 100 percent rye bread. Instead of hamburgers and hot dogs, they tracked down lamb and Spanish mackerel. Doctors told her parents that her allergies were probably related to living in Southern Florida, below sea level. So after seven years of no improvement, the family moved to Baltimore. In her teenage years, they decided to retest her, this time with 116 hypodermic injections.

"Every day for a week or so, I had to go downtown after school and get sixteen to eighteen shots," she says. "I was so skinny that one of the needles actually went through my arm and dripped on the floor. The nurse was horrified. I just laughed."

Incredibly, the tests showed no reactions to the foods that had once plagued her.

"I had either outgrown or moved away from my allergies," she writes. "I'm sorry that you were not as lucky."

Lucky. Luck is a funny thing. Most strokes of good fortune are premised on being rescued from a stroke of bad fortune. The cat has to fall out the window before he can be caught by the woman standing on a balcony below. Nobody cares when a rich man wins the lottery; it's the winner who had been on the brink of foreclosure that inspires us. My family has always spoken of my good luck in surviving reactions, and never the bad luck of having those reactions in the first place. Should I be bitter? Did I draw the genetic short straw?

When I was growing up, making those weekly trips to the allergist, the rhythm of Dr. Latkin's office never changed. We stayed with him no matter our health care plan, even when that meant periods of paying out of pocket; the continuity was comforting. We would arrive, sign in, and take our seats in the waiting room. On the floor would be the play set for the littler kids who enjoyed sliding primary-color beads along a series of loopy wire curves. The latest issues of *Highlights*, *Cobblestone*, and *Cricket* would be waiting on the low-set beech table. The walls were hung with posters displaying a collage of moments from Richard Scarry's series of Busytown picture books. Even when I last visited, less than a year ago, though the office had been renovated and repainted, the Busytown posters were still there.

As a kid, I knew Busytown from the Golden Books that my grandparents kept at their house. Richard Scarry populated his stories with anthropomorphized animals, often outfitted in traditional Swiss clothing: Blacksmith Fox, Stitches the Tailor, Hilda Hippo, and the Cat family of Daddy, Mommy, Huckle, and Sally. I use the term *story* loosely. Most of the books focused on indexing the business of daily life using the simplest of plot arcs (The Pig family is going on a train! Sally sends Grandma Cat a letter!), paced and labeled to show each step, crop, coin, switch, and gear that makes things happen.

Scarry's eye was as quirky as it was meticulous. When Jason the Mason, a pig, built a house for Stitches the Tailor, a rabbit, the illustration correctly engineered the supply of plumbing and airflow to every floor. Scarry accounted for telephone lines and labeled the sewage pipes. Depicting "moving day," Scarry detailed Stitches's quadruple-decker vehicle with scads of baby bunnies, a carrot hood ornament, a tricycle for every child strapped on top, and a paper airplane sailing out one of the car's high windows.

There is no cartoon universe better suited for an allergist's office. You could say that Richard Scarry is Bruegel the Elder for the preschool set. I'm not just basing this claim on Scarry's tendency to embed a character clothed in a blousy burlap shirt amid the populace clothed in suspenders and three-piece suits. (Though this was the kind of shirt Pieter Bruegel himself would use when attending local weddings, the better to observe his subjects. This ruse was what earned him the nickname of "Peasant Bruegel.") Coincidences of clothing aside, what I like about both are their refusal to assume an artificial focal point for the audience. These are two artists who both revel in landscapes composed of many bodies in motion.

Scarry shared Bruegel's preoccupation with—as the title of one of Scarry's books asks—*What Do People Do All Day?* In the same way that Bruegel seeded his paintings with recurring beggar figures, Scarry worked Lowly Worm into every scene, complete with his feathered Tyrolean hat, his tubular pseudo-pants, and his singular tail-shoe. Lowly is our conscience and our mischief maker. If a curtain is drawn, he'll peer over it. If a trumpet is playing, he'll hide inside of it to sing along.

The main reason Scarry's vision attracted me in childhood, just as Bruegel would fascinate me in college and ever since, is his casual and persistent depiction of life's small catastrophes. All does not go smoothly in Busytown. Lowly Worm tumbles down the air intake of a cruise ship; Mr. Frumble loses the beloved fedora that fits over his floppy porcine ears; Rudolf von Flugel, the fox pilot, downs his red German monoplane with some frequency. Houses catch fire, tractors crash, and construction workers slip and go bobbing down the river. These crises are met with the equanimity of the crowd, just as the farmer with his plow calmly ignores the flailing legs of a boy drowning at sea in Bruegel's *Landscape with the Fall of Icarus.*

This has always struck me as being the way things are, particularly if you live with illness. I don't mean to suggest that the towns we live in are callous. But as Scarry and Bruegel remind us, our towns are busy and their inhabitants preoccupied.

Once, a UVA English professor promised to introduce me to a famous poet who was reading at the university bookstore that evening. A half hour before the reading was to begin, I had an allergic reaction in the dining hall. I made it to the bookstore's bathroom, where I vomited, and then, worried I would pass out alone, lurched to the main entrance of the bookstore, where I curled up on the floor and called for help.

As one cashier hovered over me, and another dialed the hospital, my professor arrived at the bookstore with the famous poet at his side. Out of the corner of my blurry eyes, I recognized my professor—his salt-and-pepper hair, his spectacles, his sweater vest. I caught his brief pause, the murmur *Is she okay?* He did not address me by name. He acted like nothing more than a mildly compassionate stranger, one who had somewhere to be by 7 p.m. He took the poet by the elbow, and they stepped inside.

I am grateful that he kept going. Not every page is meant to tell your story. You are not the focal point of every canvas. This town is busy. And when I joined the poet's workshop a semester later, sitting in the front row of his classroom, he did not remember me from that night. So I had the chance to introduce myself as someone other than the girl with the allergies.

That's the balancing act. My job is to center on staying safe in this world, but my job is also never to assume the world should revolve around keeping me safe. We have more important things to worry about. *Don't kill the birthday girl.* The gifts are wrapped and the piñata waiting. We have a party to get to.

· · · Acknowledgments · · ·

For those looking for more information on managing food allergies, I recommend consulting the Food Allergy and Anaphylaxis Network (FAAN), the Food Allergy Initiative (FAI), and other groups mentioned in these pages.

For technical explanations and studies cited, I drew upon articles or abstracts published in the *Journal of Allergy and Clinical Immunology*, *Pediatrics* (issued by the American Academy of Pediatrics), *Mayo Clinic Proceedings*, *New England Journal of Medicine*, *Psychiatric News*, and *Annals of Allergy, Asthma & Immunology*, as well as information provided by the National Institute of Allergy and Infectious Diseases (NIAID), the European Academy of Allergy and Clinical Immunology (EAACI), and numerous mainstream news and medical resources.

In assembling the elements of science history, I am particularly indebted to *Allergy: The History of a Modern Malady*, by Mark Jackson, and Peter Duncan Burchard's research on George Washington Carver for the National Park Service.

I am grateful for the assistance and access provided by those at the National Peanut Board (Dee Dee Darden, Ryan

Lepicier, Lindsay Spencer), the Culinary Institute of America (Jeff Levine), and the American Academy of Allergy, Asthma, and Immunology (Marianne Canter, Megan Brown). I would also like to recognize the tireless and innovative research pursued by Dr. Hugh A. Sampson, Dr. Robert A. Wood, Dr. A. Wesley Burks, Dr. Gideon Lack, and their colleagues.

Thanks to the amazing team at Crown, especially my editor, Sydny Miner. Sydny, I admire your keen eye. You made this book smarter, braver, and better. Thanks as well to my acquiring editor, Heather Jackson.

Thanks to Glen Hartley and Lynn Chu of Writers' Representatives. They took a chance on a poet and have proven tireless and savvy advocates.

None of this would have happened without the Maureen Egen Writers Exchange Award from Poets & Writers, which opened the door, and the space to write afforded by fellowships to the Jentel Artist Residency Program and Virginia Center for the Creative Arts. A 2010 Individual Artist Fellowship from the D.C. Commission on the Arts & Humanities came at a critical time, and kept the roof over my head.

I had a Greek chorus of good counsel from the worlds of allergic living and creative writing, whose insights affirmed my faith in this project over and over: Maria Acebal, Natalie E. Illum, Holly H. Jones, Jenny Kales, Jennifer Kronovet, Dylan Landis, Richard McCann, Nancy McKnight, Erika Meitner, Tom Shroder, and Kate Stein. I will forever be in the debt of Meaghan Mountford, who is a reader like no other.

Nothing strikes fear into the hearts of your loved ones like the news "I'm writing a memoir!" Thanks to my friends who make cameo appearances, and in particular to Adam Pecsek for his great humor and even greater patience. Thanks to my family—Mom, Dad, Christina, Uncle Jim, my grandparents, Sara and the Jonkers clan, the Texan Beasleys, who will probably never offer me brisket again—you are all such good sports. You make this a full and lucky life.

Finally, thanks to my longtime allergist, Dr. Peter C. Latkin, and his staff. We come into your office scared. We leave smiling. You have done so much for so many.